A history of make-up

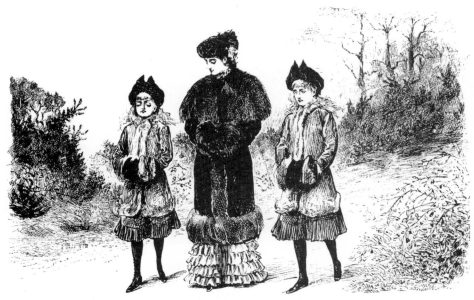

TAKING TIME BY THE FORELOCK.

Gwendoline. "UNCLE GEORGE SAYS EVERY WOMAN OUGHT TO HAVE A PROFESSION, AND I THINK HE'S QUITE RIGHT!"
Mamma. "INDEED! AND WHAT PROFESSION DO YOU MEAN TO CHOOSE?"
Gwendoline. "I MEAN TO BE A PROFESSIONAL BEAUTY!"

From *Punch*, December 1880

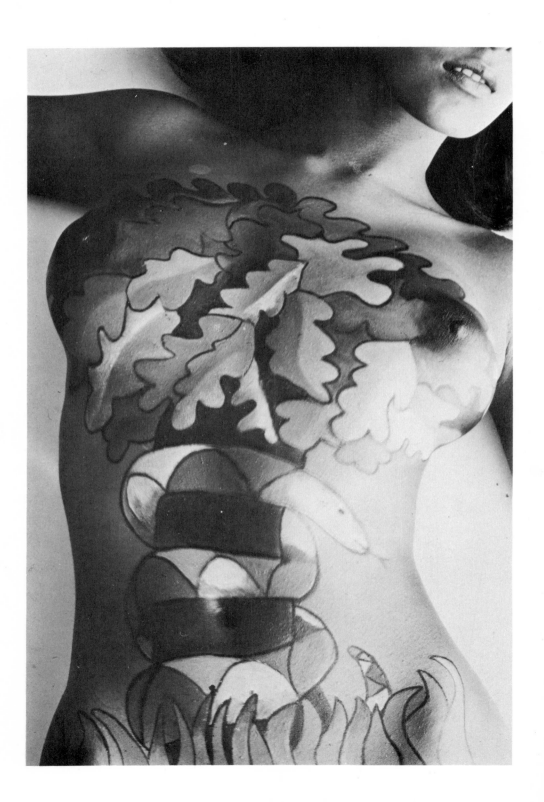

A history of make-up

Maggie Angeloglou

THE MACMILLAN COMPANY

Frontispiece
Body paint by Alan Aldridge, 1965

Library of Congress Catalog Card Number: 74-114232

First American Edition 1970
First published in Great Britain in 1970
by Studio Vista Ltd, London.

The Macmillan Company
Printed in Great Britain

Contents

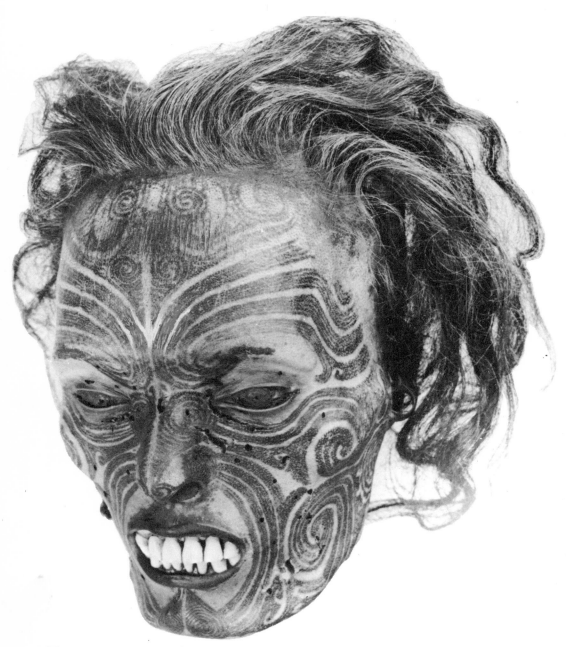

Maori mummified head. Pitt Rivers Museum, Oxford
The Maoris had a complicated form of traditional tattoo marks.

1 Paint and primitive magic

Cosmetics have held their place in public esteem with the same tenacity as religion, with which they have much in common, and as both practices lurch precariously towards the end of the twentieth century they can be compared as equally illogical, egotistical and based upon primitive necessities.

Using colour on the face is a ritual which has lost surprisingly little ground in our period, when types of make-up have altered and evolved with the speed and general acclamation of motor car designs. It is a charm against evil, as it was in the most primitive ages. The swift limning of a mouth with lipstick is usually the last thing a woman does before she steps out of the house and into the street, not with the intention of transforming herself into somebody more attractive or more colourful, but in order to make herself complete. This macabre slash of red switches a woman into her outdoor self, removing her from the safe cell of the home, and into public life. The habit of making up is so deeply ingrained that many women feel ashamed and insecure without it. 'I'm not dressed' they will say when they obviously are, but have not added the final elaboration of cosmetics.

Within the last decade it seemed as if superstition might be passing, as a more natural appearance became fashionable, and younger women appeared with bland, uncoloured faces. But old habits cling tenaciously, and the cosmetic manufacturers allied with the ancient rites to display an amazing awareness of the new cold facts of fashion, by producing the 'bare' or 'total' look which made a woman seem denuded of cosmetics simply by applying a paler colour. It is necessary to belong to a group, and immediately the younger generation equipped themselves with Identikit faces, all dewy and shining, like the Carolean vision of the happy milkmaid. And like that seventeenth-century impulse, it died away, as public reaction reproduced the face of the 1930s, when artifice was as elaborate and indiscriminate as ever in the history of cosmetics.

Cosmetics are not only barriers; they are tribal codes which are as complex and superimposed as Chinese puzzles. They are as primitive as the earliest religions, for before men had invented gods they were aware of a force of evil against which they must assume a disguise. This 'devil' haunted more sophisticated societies, as well as simple groups such as hunters and gatherers of food. It is still the 'devil' of being taken unaware that prompts the young girl to paint her face, so that she can feel prepared against any calamity of the day, even as old ladies wear clean knickers in case they are knocked down by a car. Primitive men lived in terror, and menaces were unseen and so more horrifying. Real dangers were cruel enough: they were human or animal marauders, disease or accident; but the consequences of natural disasters assured them that there were not only forces which should be placated, and which might be induced to work for man, such as gods; but that there were other and less discriminate powers which attacked the individual, and these must be avoided. They could be resisted by attack, if they were puny enemies, and this was effected by dressing in 'magic' clothes, making loud noises and painting the face to appear threatening; or they could be cheated by disguise, which entailed painting a new face on to the recognizable old one.

Warriors and priests painted the grotesque products of their imaginations on to their faces, distorting them into 'devil masks'; even children were painted in this way. Porcupines raise their quills, cats fluff out their fur, and primitive men braved the dangers of the outside world with painted faces. The men were painted because they left the compound. The safety of walls with runic charms planted and erected round an encampment or village, would scare away the evil powers; but the unfortunate men had to travel outside the enclosures to find food, and so they needed disguises. Women, who sat at home and ground corn, could be left in their natural state, they had no enemies to frighten. As more social intercourse took place, enemies were more usually other men, and they could also be terrified with incantations and masks, until they learned that certain tribes always appeared with tattooed cheeks and feather wigs . . . but even comparatively sophisticated tribesmen, who understood the intention of warpaint, might still be alarmed by the manifestation of combat. Europeans who learn judo appreciate that the cries and grunts with which the Japanese traditionally enter battle are now no more than a ritual which is consciously maintained, but even so, it is alarming.

The use of paint denoted the savage to Europeans who discovered primitive tribes, and eccentric cosmetics excited the early explorers, who added lengthy descriptions on the use of colour. La Peyère, who submitted a 'Report of Greenland' in 1647, described the Eskimos unflatteringly, as savages who were: 'sullen and untameable' and who 'painted their faces blue and yellow'.

But the study of primitive men was hardly an exact science until the first half of the nineteenth century, and the casual observations of earlier travellers reveal hardly any idea of the real nature of the savage, or even any discrimination between one race and another. The early observer was never scientifically trained, and his neglect of real facts and any minute detail about the natives he met is infuriating to readers who are accustomed to more accurate information. A typical chance discoverer was Captain Pyne. He was a captain in the renegade fleet which sailed under Prince Rupert after the English civil war, attempting to support the court of the young Charles II by piracy. Their attempts to careen their ships sometimes resulted in conflicts with native tribes, especially those which had a business arrangement to sell slaves to European merchants and who expected the Royalists to buy those unfortunate natives that they had captured and brought from the interior of Africa.

The parleys usually terminated in exchanges of shots, although arrows seem to have been more pertinent than the powder and shot of the Englishmen, who killed one native by accident and one camel by design in their action. Captain Pyne presents a curiously innocent approach to colour, for he hardly mentions pigmentation of the skin, and accepts that the baby found by the prince and brought up by him as a European was a 'blackamoor' without considering the later aspect of slavery; and reveals that one of the captains of the royal ships was a coloured African, for Captain Jacus caused a strange political involvement by running away to, and then escaping from, his own people, who fought off the attempts of the royalists to finally take the unfortunate Jacus off the shore; when he had decided to return to the fleet 'The shore was covered with the natives, who very bravely defended their coast with resolution', says Pyne. The attitudes of this plain-speaking sea captain are hardly tinged with any conceptions of race relations, and although he must have noticed the paint used in peace and in battle, he never describes it on the Africans. He did mention the colourings of the Indians when the Royalist fleet sailed westward.

Future historians would hardly have been so concise or so negligent in describing the Indians of Dominique, who welcomed the English fleet.

. . . they came to use with divers Periagos to trade, and brought us divers sorts of fruits for refreshing, which we exchanged for glass beads, and suchlike commodities. They are naturally inclined to a tawny complexion; but to avoid the stinging of the merrywings and mosquitos, they anoint their skins thick with a red paint, which they call *rockow*, in which colour they think themselves very fine; having broad and flat faces, their hair black and hard, which they wear very long, with two locks before: they bind up the rest behind like women, in which they commonly wear a macaw's or parrot's feather, with a string of fishes' teeth about their neck: some bore holes in their noses, lips and ears, in which they hang brass rings.

During the eighteenth century 'savages' were exciting curiosities who were treated like children if they were placid, or as cannon fodder if they were not. They seemed so alien to western man that he could hardly comprehend that they were human; this attitude resulted in the logical consequence of slavery. Yet to philosophers, the tribal system allied with the innocence of seeming ignorance made the painted savage a creature to esteem, he was Adam in the garden. The primitive cruelty of these men seems to have hardly impinged on the Georgians, partly because they had their own methods of barbarism, but also because paint did not frighten them. Macaronis and dandies wore powder, patches and rouge. The Indian brave was hardly more ornamented, even if his colours were cruder.

But as slavery became more widespread and desire for new territories resulted in the wholesale annexation by Europeans, the savage was increasingly degraded by more sophisticated societies. Until the eighteenth century slaves had not necessarily been black. Captain Pyne could recall an expedition to seek Prince Rupert's lost brother Maurice, who was reputedly sold into slavery by the Moors after the fleet had returned to Europe in March 1653. Any missing ship was supposed to have fallen into the hands of slave traders who sold the sailors to African monarchs or to plantation owners in the Americas. But the association of slavery with black faces ensured that natives would be regarded as subhuman, with heathen practices. The consequent 'putting down', or conversion, resulted in the elimination of many tribal traditions, including the use of paint. However, there survived two aspects of cosmetics which were supposedly primitive. The first was tattooing, which had been practised in ancient Egypt, and which travelled across several continents to reappear in Tahiti, where the crew of Captain Cook believed it was a manifestation of savagery. Cook said:

They (the Otahitians) stain their bodies by means of indentings they fill up with small instruments made of bone, cut with dark blue or blacking mixture prepared from the smoke of an oily nut . . . This operation which is called by the natives 'tattaw', leaves an indelible mark on the skin. It is usually performed when they are about ten or twelve years of age, and on different parts of the body.

9

The term 'tattaw' emerged from a native word meaning striking or knocking on wood. In his second voyage, Cook saw more tattoos which he described as 'beautiful circles, crescents, and ornaments'. Previously, in 1691, William Dampier had brought the celebrated 'painted Prince' from the southern seas to London, and Cook reiterated this raree show, by bringing Omai to London and exhibiting his tattoos; finally returning the thankful native to his home on the island of Amsterdam in the South Seas. It seemed obvious to the British that tattoo marks were synonymous with barbarisms, and yet the most superstitious men, sailors, adopted the art as their own and until the passing of sailing ships, nearly every ship of any size carried an amateur tattooist who practised his art on the crew during the long voyages. Sailors thought tattoos were good luck charms, and after the connotations with Tahiti had been forgotten, they were to become symbols of masculinity and adventure, and the young seaman regarded his first tattoo mark as a sign that he was one of the lads, so that it emerged again as a rite associated with growing up, even if it no longer took place at puberty, as it had in the South Seas. This tradition echoes the primitive belief that tattooing, like other personal decorations, is a status symbol.

Sailors could only explore the possibilities of tattoos when witchcraft was disappearing, both as a widespread cult, and as an accusation. Earlier societies, during the sixteenth century, had accepted the tattoo as the devil's mark. 'The Diuell giveth to euerie nouice a marke, either with his teeth or with his clawes,' said Reginald Scot in 1584. By 1699, a lawyer's definition was concluded by describing it as 'Stigma, or Character, and alledges that it is sometimes like the impression of a Hare's foot, or the Foot of a Rat or Spider'. Witches were marked with red spots which were similar to flea bites and with larger blue marks which were sure evidence of a witch and which had some design in them such as the outline of an animal, preferably one which was already associated with witchcraft. Dr Margaret Murray draws support from five facts for her suggestion that it was a tattoo: the colour, the actual pricking or cutting of the skin, the permanency of the mark, the pain involved, and the pressure used by the tattooist in passing his hand over the wound afterwards. This seems a reasonable supposition, and it is further strengthened by the tradition of naval tattooing, for although many patterns are used on the body there are few animal designs, and considering the sentimentality of both professions (for the sailor dreams of home and the tattooist endorses 'mother' as his perpetual message) animals would appear in the picture by logical deduction, but do not, by tradition.

Primitive men are remembered in witchcraft tattoos, and in another form of cosmetic warfare. As the necessity for disguise was emphasized, the witchdoctor emerged. In European tradition he would be the head of a coven, but in tribes he was usually a wise adviser who added reputed sorcery to his intellectual abilities in order to impress his views on the community. He would wear ritual paint, theoretically to scare the unseen forces of evil, but in time this disguise became accomplished in an ornate mask which established his dominion. In many tribes the 'devil mask' was used by warriors as well as the witchdoctor, and different masks were used for separate occasions. Finally they became ornaments to be worn on ceremonial days when a dance was to be performed, and in time they were often removed from the tribes and placed in museums and art galleries. But for a long period the mask was the most

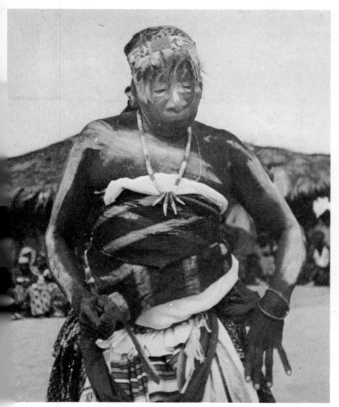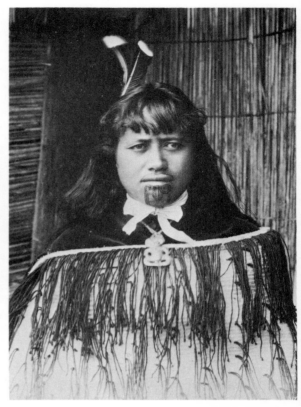

Left A woman witchdoctor, called in by the Arabesi, uses the most simple kind of facial paint.

Right The noble savage has been civilized. Wearing a neat dress and a high neckband, this Maori woman of the 1880s is a tribute to missionaries and the Victorian ethos. But a trace of the primitive is left, in wild feathers and a tattooed beard design on the chin.

necessary part of the witchdoctor's equipment, which not only disguised him from evil, and frightened human enemies, but kept his own community in a suitable state of awe. In the witch cults of Europe a similar disguise became necessary for several reasons. Initially, the leader of the coven was supposed to be a 'black man', which means dark-featured, not coloured; and a mask enabled a ruler to emerge who might be fair. The mask increased his power among the witches, for the leather shape, wreathed with horns and usually seen at night, had remarkable persuasive powers with hysterical women. Like the leather penis, it reaffirmed their illusion that they were having intercourse with a supernatural being. Finally, it disguised the warlock from any fear of discovery; it removed him from threats of blackmail, and it enabled him to continue his normal life without pursuit. Associations with the uncanny were heightened when Victorian explorers saw the masks of the tribal witchdoctors and reasoned that the same religion must implement the native tribesmen and the almost forgotten witches. Painted faces terrified the nineteenth-century mind, suggesting supernatural elements to the superstitious, and profligacy

11

to the Puritans. Even such an astute man as Charles Darwin connected paint with devils. When he visited Tierra del Fuego in 1833, the arrival of Europeans from the *Beagle* aroused great curiosity:

Several of them had run so fast that their noses were bleeding, and their mouths frothed from the rapidity with which they talked; and with their naked bodies all bedaubed with black, white and red, they looked like so many demonaics who had been fighting.

The primitive necessity to scare strangers was apparent even in the party from the *Beagle*.

Some of our party began to squint and look awry; but one of the young Fuegians (whose whole face was painted black excepting a white band across his eyes) succeeded in making far more hideous grimaces.

Aided, no doubt, by his 'disguise' face. Darwin did have the perspicacity to find out more about the composition of the Indian cosmetics, especially the white paint which must have seemed curious in a period when the cosmetic white in Europe was fatal with its charm, being mainly white lead. Darwin adds a footnote that Professor Ehrenburg of Berlin examined the substance and reported on it in 1845. When it was dry it seemed diminished, with little specific gravity. It was made up of infusoria, which are defined as minute organisms present in stagnant infusions of animal or vegetable matter; the professor added that these organisms are found in fresh water, and this was validated by the Fuegian companion on the voyage, Jemmy Button, who said that the material was found in mountain brooks. Most primitive cosmetics are made from minerals, or vegetable dyes. When Darwin visited Patagonia he found the 'giants' wore very similar marks in the same colours.

Charles Darwin was one of the few intelligent travellers who could satisfy their own curiosity and at the same time depict natives with any scientific accuracy. After the splendour of the eighteenth-century Grand Tour, many European travellers had wished to go further and see more. The increase of reliable transport and growing safety measures in areas which had been considered 'uncivilized' brought the rich men and women of the nineteenth century to within a day's march of places where traditional tribal ceremonies were still enacted; but enlightenment set in, and the religious problems of backward tribes had to be determined before they could be presented to polite society.

Meanwhile the pioneer work of observation was often done by missionaries, priests and eccentric wanderers who subsisted on hope and charity as they sought what lay beyond the Blue Ridge Mountains or at the source of the Nile. Unfortunately few of the explorers were inquisitive about small details. They could describe the paint on a warrior's face but, through lack of time, language difficulties and disinterest, had no idea what the pigment was, or where it could be found. However, they were intelligent enough to observe objectively; when James Bruce travelled to the source of the Blue Nile, he met the King of Sennar, Ismail, at a remarkable audience after the royal bath, during which Ismail kindly encouraged Bruce to rub himself with elephant grease to give him strength. It was a corrupt and decadent court and one feels that Bruce, with Scots rigour, determined that the anointment was yet another sign of permissive luxury. He did not publish an account of his journey for fourteen years, probably injured by the lack of warmth in his reception after he had produced testimony of other civilizations, where, he had noted, some tribes painted their hands and feet with yellow dye extracted from a herb called moco-moco. Coffee-house gossips were rudely disbelieving. These gentlemen adventurers were the advance guard of the pillagers. They had usually found the natives restless and disturbing. Sir Richard Burton, who eulogized the Arabs, found the Africans childish, immoral, drunken and dirty. In spite of later protestations about decadence being introduced by the white man, the African rulers were already intemperate and horrifyingly cruel when the explorers appeared.

At the same time, European knowledge of Africa was so remote that they confused gorillas with humans. The early-nineteenth-century explorers truthfully described African women who were naked but covered in grease, and found that their accuracy had been construed as licentiousness in a Mrs Grundy society. It is not surprising that Victorians became more prudent in alluding to decorations on the body. They also suffered from a glut of new experience. As each man penetrated further into the jungles of Africa or South America, he encountered more and more unusual tribes, strange habits, and unfamiliar animals. The explorers were conscious of their own importance, for as chroniclers they were awaited eagerly by Geographical Societies, Scientific Journals, the Botanical Gardens at Kew, and the American Press. Much of their information appeared piecemeal, so that tantalizing smatterings of information on rituals, marriage customs and hunting ceremonies are interspersed through narratives about the Victoria Falls or steering a boat up the Amazon. When Livingstone went to live in Africa he saw the end of the old society, perishing within his own experience, for the Africans had been terrorized and pursued by Arabs, and then by Europeans, until they fled in fear before white faces, or else they attacked strangers on sight.

The fight to save men's souls irradiates many memoirs and diaries which describe the exploration of strange countries and descriptions of inexplicable people. Many priests built a solid base of information on which anthropologists would later substantiate their findings. The early do-gooders, of the calibre of Livingstone, had to live with their converts, and the years spent in strange places leading a straitened life mellowed their attitudes to heathenism and peculiar practices. These missionaries wrote down what they saw, correctly assuming that they were doing a service to future explorers and scientists, and sometimes hoping to persuade themselves in the efficacy of their teaching. They did not necessarily portray primitive men, for it was in this way Indian customs were described by the Abbé J. A. Dubois, who lived in the early nineteenth century. *Hindu Manners, Customs and Ceremonies* delineates the different sects who paid respects to Vishnu and Siva. He describes the followers of the former god who wore an emblem on their foreheads called a namam, which consisted of three lines, one perpendicular and two oblique, forming a trident shape. The central line was red and the others were white; the mark was called after the clay used to paint on the white lines, which was namam. In Dubois's time, the white lines were disappearing and now we see a relic of the design in the red line which we associate with caste. The Hindus integrated their religion with their hygiene, appointing strict rules for bathing,

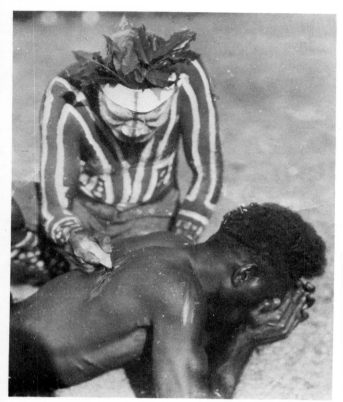
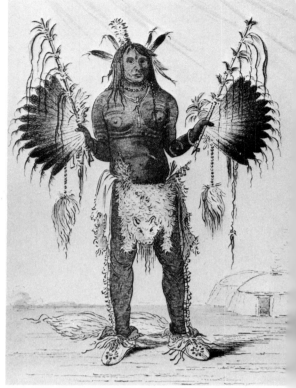

Left Initiation ceremonies in many primitive tribes include tattooing. In central Australia the elder aborigine wears full paint to perform the operation.

Right Mah-to-he-ha (The Old Bear), a warrior of the Mandan, Upper Missouri, wearing body paint.

which seemed an endless and only too unnecessary habit to the western priest; and for defecation, and for cleaning the teeth. These strict regulations on toilet had persisted virtually unaltered since the sixth century.

The Hindu namam was obviously a magic charm against evil as well as a symbol of a caste or religion. This invocation against enchantment appears throughout the world, including New Mexico, where the Jicariha Apaches have a segregated clan society called 'Striped Excrement' who are their clown figures, and who smear their faces and bodies with white clay, and then etch four black bars across their legs, face and body. This magical protection appears in a simpler version of the traditional black-bars-on-white theme in the clown of the European and North American circus ring, who has the same peculiar personality, partly innocent, wholly friendly, in his relationship with children.

Acute observance by the priest continued in North America where the French Jesuits had attempted to convert the Red Indians of Canada since the late seventeenth century. When the west was infiltrated by trappers and scouts, the priests followed, setting up crude chapels at trading posts and in frontier villages. Many religious teachers would have despaired of instructing a race which continued inter-tribal warfare after it had titularly accepted Christianity. The Jesuits were undeterred, and in each generation they continued to attempt conversions; setting up schools, trying to organize the Indian skills into profit-making concerns, in the vain hope that the tribes might cease wandering; but the Red Indians were one of the most difficult races to subjugate or restrict, depending on the historian's point of view, and they continued to fight each other and the white men, to follow buffalo and bison trails in nomadic desperation, and to execute their tribal rituals, wearing their traditional paint. They were notoriously vain, and the warriors' painted faces occupied hours of labour. They had different aspects for different ceremonies.

The backlash of the American attitude to primitive peoples hit Europe at the period when they were prepared to alter their own conceptions of savages. Livingstone's books and the tireless propaganda of enlightened explorers, combined with the beginning of a new science of anthropology, was almost reconciling the middle-class mind to painted faces and polygamy, when the fear of savages which pervaded the westerners of North America spread like fire across the country, and even influenced respectable people in Europe. The frontiersmen had reason to fear, for buffalo were disappearing, and Indians starved during cold winters; their raids on other tribes and on poorly-defended stockade towns coincided with an urge westwards among the pioneers. The Indians seem to have been more afraid of each other than of white men. They had preyed on neighbouring tribes for centuries and would hardly stop when commanded by a man of another race. Their nomadic movements alarmed the settlers for they not only never knew where the Indians were, they were also unsure who their aggressors were; and many lazy or cowardly Indians received punishment for actions by Apaches or Blackfeet. Fortunately the Indian way of life was described before the main body of the great white trek westwards, for Father Nicolas Point, writing and painting between 1840 and 1847, settled with various Indian tribes in the Rocky Mountains, and recorded their behaviour. His beautiful naïve paintings show how the Indians lived at a time when the civilization of white men had hardly impinged on them, beyond the adoption of forage caps by the more vainglorious braves. He described the race before he mentioned any particular tribe:

The skin of the Indians is the colour of copper; cheekbones are prominent; eyes are brown or black; hair is long and straight; stature is medium; legs are slim, feet are misshapen because of binding in infancy. Some distinguishing features are: canoe-men have stronger arms; hunters are more agile on their feet, have sharper vision and more adroit hands; warriors are more courageous in battle, more polished in their manners and more eloquent in their speech. Young men, on the other hand, are preoccupied with nothing but their appearance and are more vain in this respect than girls. Girls and women content themselves with separating their hair in two tresses which hang over the shoulders.

One of the Indian tribes Father Point visited on his way westward was the Kansa, and here the priest remarked on a strange habit among all primitive men, some of whom do not grow enough hair worry about it, but most of whom pluck out the beard so that the confrontation between the hairless 'savage' and the bearded civilized man was often satirical rather than illuminating.

Some of the men were occupied with plucking the hair from their faces, including the eyelashes and eyebrows. Still others were attending to their hair, an occupation they seemed to find most pleasing. Contrary to the habits of other Indians who prefer to wear their hair long, these shaved their heads, leaving only a stiffly frizzled tuft on the top. To be thus decorated was, they thought, to have the most beautiful adornment the human head could carry. . . . Soon I became aware that I, myself, was becoming the object of attention, almost the occasion for hilarity on the part of the Indian children. For some days I had given no attention to the matter of shaving. In their estimation the acme of beauty was the complete absence of hair from the chin, the eyelashes, the eyebrows, and the head. . . . If you wish a picture of the supremely self-satisfied Kansa in all his glory, you must imagine an Indian with vermilion circles about his eyes; blue, black or red streaks on his face; pendants of crockery, glass or mother-of-pearl hanging from his ears . . .

Later Father Point lived with the Coeur d'Alenes Indians, who were suffering a political coup by an illegal aspirant to the chieftainship, Stellam. This Indian Machiavelli confused the tribe by painting his body with 'bizarre figures and let[ting] it appear that he had cast a spell on the meeting'. Although the Coeur d'Alenes professed to be Christian they accepted an epidemic which broke out afterwards as proof of Stellam's magical power. Fortunately an old Indian had a vision of Christ redeeming them from sickness and he toured the camp spreading his divine message, so that Stellam's wiles were confounded. Father Point believed that the hallucination was the result of the shock caused by Stellam's attempted necromancy, or the delirium of sickness. Whatever the reason, the hypnotic influence of body-painting had affected the tribe.

Father Point noticed a cadet branch of the Blackfeet, the Fisheaters, with 'their costumes and visages each one stranger and more picturesque than the other'. He also visited a lodge belonging to a notable of the tribe and remarked that along with the ornamented calumnet (the totem peace-pipe carried into battle) there was a bowl of perfumed water, for the Indians were not considered dirty by those who lived with them, although they repelled the sensitive white nostril by the smell of animal fat which they smeared on their hair and bodies. As travellers journeyed further south on the American continent they discovered ornamental traits among southern tribes, which were similar to those of the Red Indians and tribes on other continents. The narrow distinction between Red Indian and Mayan customs is typified by the bead swinging from a braid, which is placed before the eyes of a young Mayan boy, so that he develops a squint. The Indian custom of carrying babies on the back by tying them to a board is extended in the ancient Mayan custom of lashing babies to a board so that the head will be elongated. However the Mayans seem solitary in their tradition of filing their teeth to sharp points and then inlaying them with semi-precious stones such as turquoises and jade. Like the Tahitians they followed the ancient Egyptian practice of tattoos, and like some African natives they cut their skin into decorative patterns. The habit of mutilating in order to attract appears throughout the world, for Australian primitives removed their teeth, Eskimos perforated their lips and cheeks and other tribes, including our own, made holes in ears or noses.

At the end of the nineteenth century most of the world which could be traversed suffered from tourists. The more recondite tribes, such as the head-hunters in South America or the pigmies in Africa, moved away from these boundaries of civilization which were defined by tracks, mission houses and trading posts. The anthropologist arrived, and occasionally he was too late to save the ornaments of a dying tradition. In some areas the natives were assimilated equally into the general population, in others they became the servants and farm workers of white settlers. Many tribesmen went into the towns, contending with a commercial society by working to earn money. Warpaint, or the cosmetic art of warning real and imaginary enemies, had no place in a community in which men wore trousers and bowler hats, and women covered their breasts with blouses. The impression generally held of tribesmen was that they were dirty, lazy and slow to adapt to the accepted mores of western civilization. In fact primitive peoples accepted the habits of their new masters only too swiftly, and within three generations the world of magic and painted faces had retreated, or had been lost. Older civilizations escaped lightly, for many Europeans were in awe of their traditions. The Arabs and the Asians retained many of their caste and social customs, and because of their romantic and ancient associations the red mark of the Hindu or the veil worn by Moslem women was regarded with reverence. Arabic cosmetics were not worn to terrify, which made them acceptable, and they had no effeminate connotations to most Victorian writers, except Charles M. Doughty, who described the Bedouin tribesmen in 1876, when he was the guest of Zeyd, a sheik of the Fejir Bedouins. Doughty recounts:

In all Arabia both men and women, townsfolk and Bedouins, where they may come by it, paint the whites of their eyes blue, with kahl or antimony; thus Mohammed Ibn Rashid has his birdlike eyes painted. Not only would they be more love-looking, in the eyes of the women, who have painted them and that braid their long manly sidelocks; but they hold that this sharpens too and will preserve their vision. With long hair shed in the midst and hanging down at either side in braided horns, and false eyes painted blue, the Arabian man's long head under a coloured kerchief, is in our eyes more than half-feminine; and in much they resemble women.

2 Cosmetics in the ancient civilizations

Cosmetics continued to have religious significance after the establishment of systems of government. Tribes formed and re-formed to constitute nations with defined territories, and cults of nationalism replaced those of villages. Identification was extremely important to these new societies, whose members had dim memories of a time when they were nomadic, with no buildings, no class stratifications and no defined trades or interests with which they might associate, except the most primitive group, the family, which had extended to embrace the village, the city, the district and the nation. Ritual engineered the lives of comparatively sophisticated people as well as less intelligent serfs and slaves; and governments understood that the religion of their people had an important influence in their own methods of administration. Terror had receded, for men became less nervous of unseen forces when they could harness waterpower or build fairly solid dwellings which they could barricade against real or imaginary enemies. The power of early religions lay in mystery. The witchdoctor was replaced by the priest, who not only had strong political power, but also surrounded himself with an aura which though less crude than the feathered robe and horrific mask of tribal men, nevertheless established his domination, and the dominion of his gods, in the minds of the people. Religions had codes which would sublimate different aspects of human experience; some preached rebirth, others predestination and fortitude in suffering; but most of them concentrated on the great inexplicable happening, death. The Egyptians in particular enclosed death in its own mummy case of ritualistic significance. In these rites, cosmetics added indispensable magic.

The 'civilized' Egyptians did not invent their own cosmetics. They had a tradition which can be traced to the mesolithic period (10000 to 5000 BC) when the future nation was composed of hunters and shepherds living in the valley of the Nile, who smeared their bodies with grease and oil from the castor plant, and who had tattoo marks on their faces and bodies. When the early Egyptians settled to an agricultural way of life, in about 3500 BC, they developed cosmetics as protection against the sun; among the remains of their villages, archaeologists have found eyepaint ground from green malachite on schist palettes, and cleansing oils of wild castor plants. Even in this primitive period there are indications that ointments and perfumes were bartered from one area to another; in a wall painting in the tomb of Khum-hotep at Beni Hasan there are illustrations of visitors carrying eyepaint as a gift for the dead dignitary, who was the governor of the eastern desert.

By 5000 BC eyepaint had become quite sophisticated although only two colours were available. Black antimony powder was used to etch in the shape of the eyebrows. The black lines which shaped the eyelids and which extended over the side of the face in 'wings' were drawn in galena which was an early type of kohl, composed of a form of lead ore. The green make-up was the most famous unguent used in ancient Egypt. It was always reputed to be made of

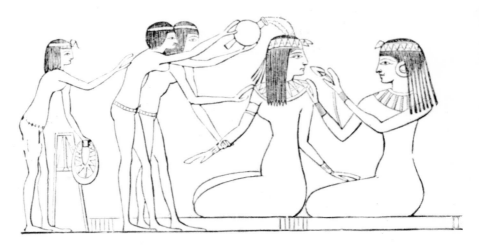

An Egyptian Lady at her Toilet vase painting, c. 1400 BC
The perfuming of an Egyptian lady, attended by maids whose dress is hardly more
elaborate than her own.

malachite until a revelation in the early 1920s suggested that no malachite
was available in any of the territory inhabited by the early Egyptians; as the
green eye ointment appears in very early remains it could either be that the
Egyptians had trading relationships with other countries while they were
still at the agricultural stage, or that there had once been malachite in Egypt
which was played out.

This paste was not primarily ornamental. The grotesquely exaggerated
designs on the stylized Egyptian face are not restricted in sex, age or class;
for like their very earliest forefathers, the Egyptians needed paste on their eyes
to protect them from the sun; and while it may appear strange that wall paintings show quite young children with lurid make-up on their eyes, the truth is
that careful parents would superintend this cosmetic peculiarity as a precau-
tion. One of the ingredients was hydrosilicate of copper and this was an
immediate remedy for suppuration caused by glare. Fashionable Egyptians
also etched their eyes in with a mixture of ants' eggs pounded in a mortar,
which seems to have been a purely ornamental ointment.

Hairstyles had more than a decorative function. The Assyrians developed
fashions in hair to the exclusion of nearly every other cosmetic art, oiling and
perfuming it, and trailing long sideboards down their cheeks. Their faces were
shaved, but the actual beard, with a neatly clipped line on the jaw which
appears to be allied to the art of topiary, it is so like a clipped yew, was grown
down over the chest in layers of ruffles, like the front of an exquisitely ironed
and tucked shirt. Their court ceremonials prescribed certain types of formal
coiffures according to position and employment. The Egyptians also attached
symbolism to the growth of hair: along the stretches of North Africa it suggested
masculinity and strength.* As court ceremonial became rarified to an un-
precedented degree, the Egyptians used false beards in lieu of real ones, especially in a period when many men were clean-shaven; and when Queen
Matshrtpdont ruled, she wore a stylized ceremonial fake beard, which was

*As it did among the Israelites, the belief being incarnated in the story of Samson, and subsequently
reinforced by it.

19

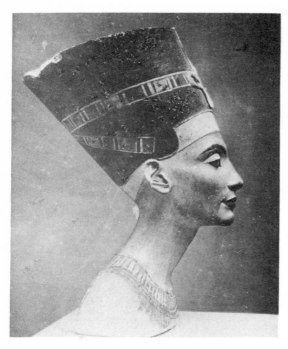

Plaster head of Queen Nefertiti, *c.* 1400 BC. Staatliche Museen zu Berlin

gilded, and which she could adopt in council or during ceremonies when she had to assert that she could be as authoritative as a man. This illusion of masculine power and the bearded lady seems to have trailed into our own traditions with the whispered superstition among her contemporaries that Queen Elizabeth had a beard.

The upper classes of the Nile would spend many contemplative hours at their make-up, but their hair probably merited as much attention as the whole of the rest of the body. Plaiting those intricate little braids which were bushed to make a great blue-black head-dress must have occupied a sunlit afternoon. In time even the most vain Egyptians succumbed to the easy expedient of using false hair, and finally wigs, which conveyed a greater impression of power than they could have borne with their own hair. The wig became as stylized as the beard, until it was translated into a great golden head-dress for the pharoahs, and so immortalized by its reproduction on the mummy figures.

Egyptian hairdressers were incredibly skilled. Even allowing for the artificiality of the wig, they appear to have cut the hair in careful tiers so that the head of a fashionable courtier was as neatly geometric as the pyramid, and somewhat similar. Women used their heads as an aid to general charm. Before the introduction of the ceremonial wig, or in the comparative informality of private homes, they braided flowers into their hair, and secreted perfumed balls into it near the scalp and during the hours spent dining or talking with equally cosmeticized guests, the balls melted, and runnels of perfume slowly seeped through their plaits, or the perpetually popular chignons.

The use of perfume had at first been restricted to the priests. It was originally one of the perquisites associated with death, for the art of perfumery, like so many other cosmetics, can be traced to the Egyptians, and for them scents and unguents were irrevocably associated with the mystery of death. Many of the creams, ointments and perfumes which we use today and which are advertised by manufacturers as renewing youth or adding vitality, originated in the ceremony of mummification. The oils were refined from those early experiments with castor pods which had protected the naked bodies of hunters from the sunlight. The Egyptians had particular affection for flowers, and they added these to their ointments in an attempt to make some preservative which would not only cocoon the mortal body, but would keep it as wholesome-smelling as any clean-living Egyptian aristocrat would wish to be in life.

The process of mummification was not only advanced, but also well organized; for as the Egyptian priests prepared for the eventuality of death with such zest, it could be put into operation with the alacrity of a modern, highly powered military manoeuvre, and was swifter and more efficient than many funeral parlours. Immediately the death of a ruler, such as Tutankhamen, had been made public, the nation went into mourning with ceremonial cries of agitation followed by silence and fasting. The men of the court stopped shaving, and this ritual would continue until the burial. Over seventy days were occupied in preparing the body for its translation to the tomb, and during this time the finest products of the period were collected to be buried with it: linen scarves and wrappers, the best vintages of wine, and most important of all, the forty-three jewelled objects which would be wrapped into the folds of the mummy cloth. Ointments and perfumes were bottled into alabaster jars for the future use of the dead king, with a wig case, mirrors and cosmetics. Unfortunately, although traces of these were found when the tomb of Tutankhamen was excavated, they were unstoppered when the archaeologists came to them and so the contents had evaporated, or they had been disturbed by the unscrupulous local people who thieved from the tombs before the arrival of the professionals; and in fact, soon after the internment. However, many other mummies show the glimmerings of long-lasting make-up and calculations can be made about the material which was missing. The most interesting surgical developments took place as aids to mummification, in which the brain was drawn out through the nostrils and the skull dissolved in aromatic ointments. The organs were removed by an operation on the side of the body, and then the hollow was filled with cassa and myrrh and aromatics, after a wash of palm wine. The organs were embalmed and placed in small urns to accompany the mummy. By now the body was simply a shell which was shaved clean and put into natron, a hydrated carbonate of sodium which is found on the shores of inland lakes. This absorbed any dampness or humidity left in the carcase. After seventy days the body was removed and placed on a tall bier. The mummifiers then bandaged it, carefully distinguishing so that no part of the skin touched another, each finger was bound separately while ointments were poured on to the corpse and prayers were recited. In the case of Tutankhamen, the unguents were probably used too liberally and contributed to the decomposition of the body, so that finally only the sections which were gilded escaped decay. Into the layers of fine linen was tucked the generous assortment of jewels to help the dead man on his way.

This lengthy diversion on mummification and the remains of the royal tomb in the ancient kingdom of Thebes, demonstrates the peculiar myths which surrounded the early cosmetics. But it was not surprising that the unguents could not remain the secret of the priests. Not only were they an interesting black market commodity, but they also became a trading weapon with adjacent nations, as ointments and perfumes travelled about the Mediterranean following the fashions of the time. Our knowledge of the perfumes comes from Pliny, who lived in the time of Christ, but who recorded those potions which

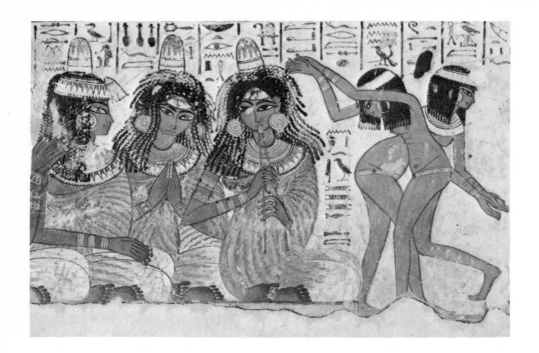

had captivated the ancient world. Mendes, in Egypt, was a notable centre for perfumery and to it came the raw essences culled in other countries; markoram from Cos, the home of the celebrated Coan Quince Cream which was used by fashionable ladies to smooth their complexions; saffron from Rhodes; rose-water from Phaselis; panther, an exotically-named essence from Tarsus, and, most potent and long-lived of all, from Cyprus came chypre, the musky scent which is still used in perfumery today.

Many of the middle eastern cosmetics passed through Egypt even if they did not originate there, for the priestly tradition established an industry which ensured that refinements and experiments would be carried out there, even when the final product would travel back to source. The most influenced society was that of the Romans, who relied upon subjugated Egypt to manufacture cosmetics and scents which they could not produce themselves. Because of this mastery over beauty, a sinister aura adhered to the Egyptians, which endowed them with magical knowledge, and which probably resulted in their reputation as 'gippos', the secret society with supernatural abilities. The hypnotic effect of Egypt was to be immortalized in Roman legends in the figure of Cleopatra. She became an idea rather than a reality, and her subtlety was enhanced by a use of make-up which must have seemed outrageous to the Romans of her time. The Egyptians were not afraid of colour, unlike other civilizations condemned to heat they wore brilliant robes, hung about with jewels. This attitude to adornment dictated the mode of dress throughout society, for even the dancing girls, who wore nothing else at all, would have collars of lapis lazuli and gold. Egyptian fashions emphasized this passion for gold, as in the second millenium women wore tight corsages, laced to thrust their breasts outwards and to display their brazenly gilded nipples or blue-painted veins. Cleopatra experimented with eye colours to effect, using black galena on the eyelid and to delineate her brows, and painting the upper lids deep blue, and the lower lids bright green.

Upper-class ladies carried all their cosmetics in a toilet box, and one of these intricate cases exists in the British Museum. It belonged to Thuthu, the wife

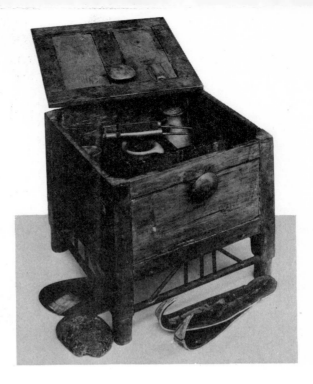

Banquet scene from the tomb of Nebamun at Thebes, *c.* 1400 BC. British Museum, London

Thuthu's toilet box, *c.* 1300 BC. British Museum, London

of Ani, and many of its contents would make attractive additions to cosmetic boxes of our own time. Make-up was a slow operation so she had special slippers in the case, as well as more sturdy sandals, and elbow cushions on which she could find a steady base from which to pivot her arms when she outlined her eyes. Pumice stone was included to remove body hair, as well as to smooth the rough skin on her knees and elbows. Eye pencils were kept in a special tube, and were made of wood or ivory, to use for the shadow powder which could be utilized in damp or humid weather; and there was a liquid colour which was also an ointment, and which would shield her eyes from the glare of the sun. A bronze dish was included, and in this she would mix her own colours, adjusting them to suit her taste and the occasion. The three cosmetic pots are empty but one can imagine that they held ointments and face creams, and that they would be similar to other analysed Egyptian cosmetics which have been found intact, and still scented, and which contain one part perfumed resin to nine parts animal fat. These complicated cosmetics were known in other areas. At Ur a lipstick was found which is probably four or five thousand years old. In Scythia the women painted their faces, and Pliny mentions a Scythian scent named after one of the great kings of the past which was made of extraordinary fusions of balm, honey, crocus, lotus and vine as well as aromatic herbs. It was related to those mysterious Egyptian scents.

These perfumes were originally made from burnt resin and scented woods, which have endured to our own age in the perpetually utilized and pervasive sandal. They were largely antiseptics as well as unguents and the whole craft, as secretive as any medieval guild tradition, was originally practised in chambers off the main temples which were private to the priests. They wrote their secret recipes on the walls of these small darkened rooms. The hypnotic effect of scented air during religious ceremonials was appreciated even at that time, and the idea was carried to Israel by Moses to become part of a religious tradition which was to extend into the Christian faith.

In later centuries a puritan northern superstition claimed that the races of

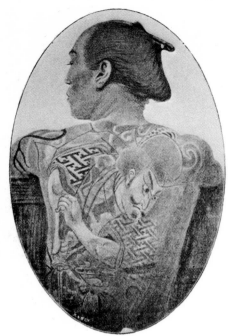

Japanese tattoo,
late nineteenth century

the Middle East perfumed themselves to cover the heavier and more irritating smells of dirt and sweat, but the Egyptians, like several other early civilized peoples, were almost paranoiac about personal cleanliness. This cult of the bath culminated in special 'unguent' rooms with a ceremonial addition of body oils which they deduced must preserve the living body from the problems of age and sun, as well as they did the dead. They washed before and after meals, and their lengthy showers were prefaced with a rough rub-down with sand which was intended to clean the pores, and which was followed by complete washing down. Most races desire complexions which are not their own, but the Egyptians were pleased with their own tanned skins, and the women made little attempt to alter them, except for the use of a ritualistic make-up for certain ceremonials when they painted their faces with ceruse, the first appearance of the cosmetic which was to remain unaltered until the end of the nineteenth century. They also evaded wrinkles by using face masks of egg white.

Inevitably the more fashionable Egyptians appreciated that cosmetics were rather more than sun-visors, and during the reigns of Rameses and the Ptolemies, they experimented with different types of eye shadows, adding purple and blue to the repertoire, and utilizing the natural ores of the country to make the pigments, which were the same as those used in their pottery and their wall paintings. Ochre was used to colour their cheeks, and carmine on the mouth.

Tattooing was extended to a skilled craft by the Egyptians. Previously, the primitive scars on the faces and the body of tribesmen had been less ornamental than signs of adherence to a group, added in the same spirit as the brand marks of cattle. The careful modern method of puncturing the skin with a needle or some other similar instrument and then injecting a dye under the skin appeared in the Nile Valley between 4000 and 2000 BC. During these centuries the craft spread in a complicated pattern across the world, and historians have traced the tattoo to Crete, Greece, Persia and Arabia under the third and fourth dynasties (2800 BC – 2600 BC), and then across southern Asia to the area south of the Yangtze-kiang in China. This would be in about 2000 BC. From there it was taken to Japan by the Ainu, a migrant tribe who developed a religious respect for the tattoo and considered that the craftsman had a divine gift. The Shans took the tattoo to Burma where it also had a religious significance. The Japanese also considered that it was ornamental and it was perhaps this secular reaction to the aura of divinity about the craft which enabled the Japanese to develop new designs and to perfect the ornamental aspect of the tattoo until they were considered the great masters when the Europeans adopted tattooing again. From Japan, the areas of Formosa, Borneo, the Philippines and other Pacific islands cultivated the idea; and the Polynesians, a race which moved from India at about 400 BC, carried their own tattoo designs to New Zealand. It went north too, with the Romans, who added new techniques to the primitive blue skin markings already practised by Ibernians, Celts and Teutons.

The Japanese had other cosmetic aids during the same period as the Egyptian culture; during their neolithic period, between 4500 and 2500 BC, the Joman tribe had a rite which probably entailed removing teeth and filing them down. In the remains of both men and women from the ages of seventeen or eighteen, the canines and the incisors are removed, and the small pottery figures of the same age have distinct tattoo marks on their bodies. By the Bronze and Iron Ages in Japan, as elsewhere, mirrors of polished metal were buried with the dead, a fairly conclusive proof that the living were interested in their own appearance. In later centuries the Japanese discovered paint, and in tomb sculptures of the third century AD the mourners have highly cosmeticized faces, which would have shown the proper attitude to grief, with the same determined set-piece and colour formula as that which was developed later for the formalized characterization of the Japanese or the Italian theatre. By this period the tattoo was relinquishing its fashionable role, and the permanent dyes were probably replaced by an infusion of black soot. The tattoo at one time replaced the brand as the permanent stigma of a criminal in Japan.

The Myceneans had the same preoccupation with cleanliness as the close-neighbouring Egyptians, and they developed their own perfumed oils and unguents; boiling coriander, ginger grass, wine and honey, into ointments which were then potted into exquisite alabaster jars. These occupied places in their graves, where there were alabaster spoons used to dip into the cream, as well as tweezers of bronze which were found with the body of a man, displaying that interest in hairlessness which then permeated tribal and civilized men.

It is a demonstration of the Egyptian interest in design and in ostentatious displays of wealth, that the containers and implements of beauty were more carefully manufactured than the cosmetics. The ointments and pigments were probably generally used by all higher strata of society and so the Egyptian noble exhibited his individual splendour in gold pots, jewelled spatulas with which to apply his eye shadow, wig boxes, and decorated mirrors. Ultimately they ended with him, as visas for life after death, which evinced his taste and his superior riches. The young Tutankhamen, whose tomb displays an astonishing plethora of information on life and manufacture of his time, was only about nineteen when he died. His tomb was not only a monument to him but to the exaggerated grief of a nation which had developed new art forms during his short reign. In it, pots of unguents were found, scattered higgledy-piggledy in the dark side-chambers. Finally, these pathetic relics, and the uncertain memories of later writers, were to commemorate the first sophisticated cosmetics.

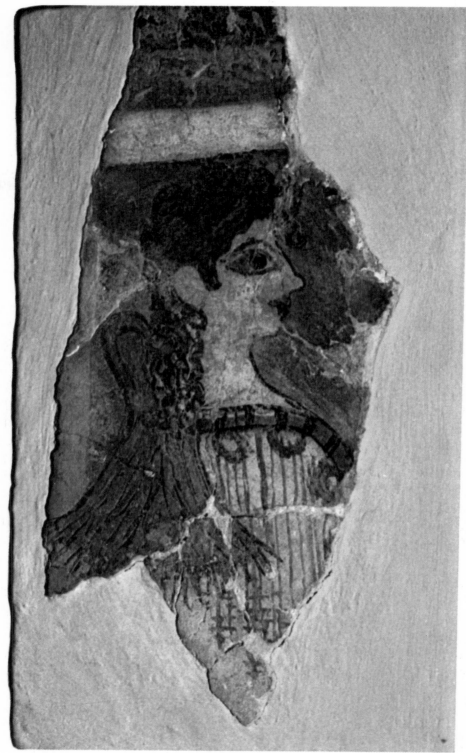

La Parisienne c. 1550-1450 BC. Heraclion Museum, Crete
This head has its affinities with those of the late-nineteenth-century ladies who appear in the paintings of Renoir or Manet; self-assured, elaborately coiffured, and with a slash of poppy colour on the lips which was not completely honest.

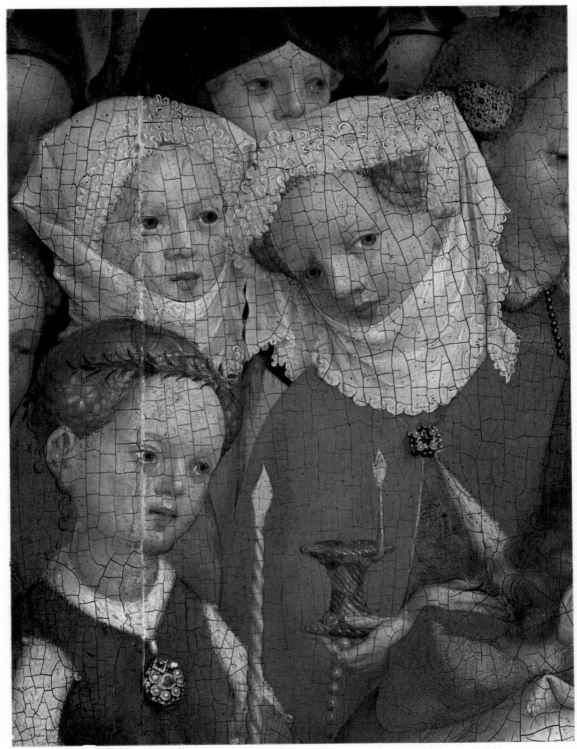

Stephen Lochner *The Presentation in the Temple* 1447. Detail. Hessisches
Landesmuseum, Darmstadt. The late medieval face is usually a white egg. Stephen
Lochner gave his women soft transient complexions, but although their eyebrows
are plucked they are innocent of cosmetics.

3 Greece and Rome; and eastern attitudes

Unlike the Romans, who assimilated ideas on make-up from Egypt, the Greeks had a stoic attitude to cosmetics which resulted in a halt in their development. One might even suggest that this termination of progress continued until our own century, for certainly no remarkable additions were made to the repertoire of the Egyptian priests or their heirs, the so-called necromancers. The Greeks had little time for more languorous pleasures during their early history, and when their society became established and wealthy it was dominated by an ideal of masculinity, which had a tradition of hardiness. They certainly knew of the unguents of Egypt, and many Roman writers mention Greece as the source of perfumes and cosmetics, although probably these were basically Egyptian, and the recipes had been preserved in Greece. Jars and pots have been excavated with remnants of perfumed creams inside; and these are often beautifully executed suggesting that, as in Egypt, the container could be more important than its contents.

Both the Greek and Roman cultures had bridging contact with Egypt through the Cretans, who used a whitener on their skins, and underlined their eyes; and the Etruscans, where the women had equal status with the men, and who produced a type of beauty much admired in Greece. A certain neatness in design about their depictions of women suggests carefully coiffed hair and manicured hands and feet. The Etruscans in particular left incontrovertible proof of their interest in make-up, in the shape of mirrors, boxes and flasks, and utensils for nails, or spatulas with which they applied their rouge.

But in Greece women were supposedly chattels, although some of them seem to have had enough personality to intrude into the masculine society. However, the male was the perfect creature and he had the right to baths which were taken in public bath-houses, and which were advanced to running water, carried by pipes through tubs made of earthenware and polished stone, or even of silver.

The respectable housewife had no opportunity to use colour on her face. Men, seduced by the habit of using oils and perfumes on their skins after their baths, probably experimented with rouge and lip salve; and it has been suggested that the young boys who flourished in the homosexual society might have been painted; but the Greek ideal was basically concerned with purity and they seem to have found physical grace more attractive if it was absolutely natural. However the Greek man also turned to courtesans, and it was through these that the craft of make-up was preserved in Greece. In the *Phaedrus*, Plato suggests what many reasonable men must have felt at that time, that 'there are some animals... in which nature has mingled a temporary pleasure and grace in their composition. You may say that a courtesan is hurtful, and disapprove of such creatures and their practices, and yet for the time they are very pleasant.'

As in Victorian society, the woman at home was not expected to be pleasurable, her work was to direct the house and bear the children and her choice

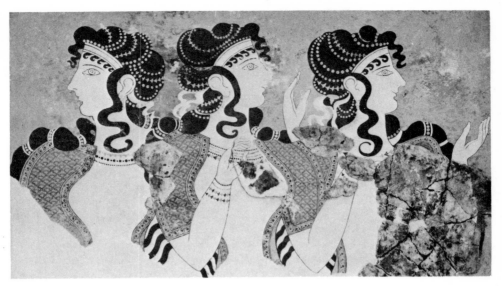

The Three Ladies c. 1600 BC. Palace of Knossos, Crete
Cretan women created a pattern in make-up in the northern Mediterranean. Their hair was carefully bound and their eyes were painted in the same manner as those of Nefertiti.

was arranged by business discretion; but the courtesan had the imagined allure of mystery which was to survive to later periods. The toilet of the rich Greek courtesan was even recorded:

Her slaves massaged her from head to foot before placing her in a scented bath; she was then caressed with swan's feathers so as to dry the parts of her body which were still damp. Then, she was rubbed with perfumed oils brought from the Orient. A depilatory was then carefully applied. Her hair was washed, perfumed and pomaded before being plaited. Her coiffure was completed with filigree braid, and gold and silver lamé ribbons. A black coating touched up her eyebrows and the edges of her eyelids were drawn with a brush dipped in incense black. Her eyes were underlined with kohl.

A knowledgeable courtesan had another trait, she would perfume her breath by carrying scented liquid in her mouth and rolling it about with her tongue.

Face colour was always peculiarly compounded, and the Greek heterae would rouge with puperissium, a root from Syria which was macerated in vinegar. Ceruse was used to whiten skin. But the puritan attitude of men towards these dangerous practices was summed up by Lucien, a writer at the end of the second century who said sourly: 'If one could see women getting out of bed, one would find them even less attractive than monkeys.'

The only exception allowed to the decorous rule was in the treatment of hair. Perhaps the sanctity of hair had been established by the ancient goddesses, whose hair undulated like the sea; it could be dyed, and dyed hair was actually accepted as necessary for mourning when it was darkened. It could also be reddened, or made blonde. This is the first indication of the tradition which was maintained by the Latin races and later by western society, that fair hair is more desirable than black and has connotations of innocence, superior race and sexual desirability. The blondes of ancient Greece were induced by a pomade of yellow flower petals, a potassium solution, or other coloured powders which veiled their hair with red, gold or silver. In memory of those mother-figure goddesses, it could be curled with tongs and braided into designs which were touchingly elaborate compared with the sparse decoration otherwise allowed to women.

In spite of the little information left on Greek cosmetics, it is obvious that the Romans culled their ideas on make-up, as on more important aspects of social life. Rome was a jackdaw culture.

When in 129 BC the Romans had conquered the great Phoenician city of Carthage they were the virtual rulers of the civilized world. At this moment of world supremacy the character of the actual Romans subtly altered, and the new effete regime seemed to be inheriting the glory of the ancient city but eliminating at the same time those patrician qualities of which the Romans boasted. A simple race, the Romans were suddenly inundated by new wealth, new relaxation and new languor. Their situation was the common satirical one of the foolish man who wins the football pools; they were determined to enjoy all their new sensations at once; their slaves often came from more sophisticated nations than their own, and many Romans, determined on establishing their status and influence, must have glanced over their shoulders falteringly at the ghosts of the Etruscans, the Greeks, and the seemingly decadent Egyptians. The old class system had gone, and corruption had taken its place, for the nobility controlled the Senate and the equality of Roman citizens was annulled in 194 BC. There were increasing demands for luxuries which had only been revealed to the Romans when they encountered the Greek culture in Asia Minor. Two hundred years before the birth of Christ, the Romans were devouring, but not digesting, all the habits of the Hellenic and oriental peoples which they had conquered. They consulted fortune tellers, they attempted to divine the future from entrails and the stars, they privately worshipped Bacchus with resulting orgies, poisonings and legal disputes. As the upper classes became more despotic and decadent, the lower classes were pacified with circuses.

Among these new luxuries, cosmetics appeared.

The bath was a male pursuit, as it had been in Greece, and the public baths no doubt arose from a memory of those tubs of silver through which the water eternally flowed. The Romans had the money, the inclination, and the inventiveness to establish a bathing system which has never been bettered. When a Roman entered the bath-house he was greeted and led to a changing room, where he removed his clothes, leaving them with a slave. He then went into a tepid room and bathed, accustoming his body to the heat; the second chamber was a sweating room where he would sit on a bench and talk to friends, occasionally sprinkling water on his body when the heat became unbearable; this room must have been as awesome and exclusive as a gentlemen's club in London during those years when real power was centred over the port bottle, and national decisions could be made from a leather chair in a window bay. The final room was for massage, the body was rubbed with oil after the skin was toned with a scraper. This ritual had evolved from the customary preparation for battle which the Greeks had appreciated before the Romans. As such, it had a suggestion of doom, a meticulous concentration on oiling the physical mechanism to detract from the consideration of death. It had been a grim performance in the past; but in Rome it had become a social perquisite, and elaborate baths were built into private houses.

As in many over-sophisticated cities, men and women led their own separate lives. It is true that Roman women did not have the emancipation of women of our own day, but they did have a certain political power through influence, and they had their own circles of friends in which they could play games of love-making, jealousy and connivance. Unlike the Greek women, they could not be used with authority, and so there was no submission to the men's dictates on cosmetics; as the slaves became more numerous and the riches of colonies poured into the city, there was competition to see which family could win in the race of ostentatious expenditure—and one consequence was that the matriarchs had time on their hands.

Hair was the most important aspect of beauty, partly because of the male assumption that this was the most discreet token of femininity. Writing in the second century, Apuleius expresses the Roman attitude in *The Golden Ass* when he says that the first thing he notices in a pretty woman is her hair, shining with gold light and glossy with spikenard lotion. Although he spares a glance for the dark-haired woman, for him the truly attractive girl has blonde hair. The Romans debased his view, dyeing their hair red or blonde with a soap from Germany which had originated in Gaul. Blonde hair became the brand of a prostitute. The savages of the north traded with the Romans, and sent this unguent, rolled into balls, to the Roman perfumers. They also sent the fair hair of their women, which was made up into ornate wigs. Roman cheeks were stained vermilion, and the skin was whitened with a chalk powder.

As the Roman desire to ape the Greeks extended to make-up, they hardly progressed beyond the ideas which the Asian Greeks had assimilated during their observance of more eastern races; and with this impact of Arabic cultures, came the return of the Egyptian products. The Egyptians themselves had become reconciled to being a second-rate power, in that they had assiduously turned their attention to those pleasures they had always favoured in the past, but which had been neglected in the years when they had played power politics up and down the Mediterranean. They grew flowers, and turned the essences into perfumes, including one which was called 'Egyptian' by contemporaries, even as the pervasive chypre was named after Cyprus. Oris was another favourite which has survived to our own day and which was made of the dried root of irises, which smelt of violets. Hilcesies in *On Materials*, describes the splendours of the Egyptian perfumes, as seen by the Greeks and Romans:

Some perfumes are rubbed on, others are poured on. Rose perfume is used for a drinking party, also myrrh and pumice; the last is wholesome and good for patients suffering from a lethargic fever. Scent from dropwort is wholesome and keeps the brain clear. Scents of marjoram and tufted thyme are suited for a drinking party, and also saffron crocus if not mixed with too much myrrh. Gilliflower scent is fragrant and very helpful to digestion.*

A Greek writer, Antiphanes, in *Thorikan Villagers, or Digging Through* depicts the bath of the period:

> She's really bathing! well then, what!
> Yes, she's got a box inlaid with gold and from it
> She anoints her feet and legs with Egyptian scent,
> Her cheeks and nipples with palm oil, one of her arms
> With bergamot-mint, her eyebrows and her hair
> With sweet marjoram, her knee and neck
> With scent of tufted thyme.*

*translation, Jack Lindsay

The Egyptians still used their dramatic face paint which electrified the Romans, daubing their eyes with galena and malachite, and staining their cheeks with red ochre in the same manner as the Arabs. The poor fellahin still anointed their bodies with castor oil extract like their naked forefathers, but the upper income groups had already devised cunning ways to render oils and fats into perfumes by soaking flower petals in oil. The habit of staining the hands and feet with henna was also translated to Rome.

During the periods of Greek and Roman asceticism, there had been a diminishing interest in cosmetics for men, but as the apparent decadence of the Romans increased, the citizens who had stopped short of anything beyond a hot steam bath, began to curl their hair where it lay on their shoulders, and to use perfume. Extremists added rouge and face whiteners, and even the occasional beauty patch.

In the two centuries before and after Christ, Latin writers amused their audiences with satires, criticisms and odes in which they assured their mistresses that their beauty was rather owing to artifice than to nature. As in most fairly sophisticated societies, these idealists preached a revolt against cosmetics which actually appears in retrospect as a defence of them, for they accepted wigs, perfumes, rouges and hair dyes as necessities. The blonde hair which had been the prostitute's mark appeared in the most aristocratic circles, especially after the retinue of Messalina had imported German wigs to wear on grand occasions. One of the most severe critics of cosmetics was Lucretius who died fifty-five years before the birth of Christ and who castigated the new tone in public life which was already making more sober and plain-speaking Romans uneasy. To men like him, the younger people seemed unlikely heirs to the splendour of the old city, as they wandered about the city, playing obscene practical jokes, painting their faces and changing from one ensemble to another. Memories of the dreaded Nero and Caligula perpetually haunted the older generation, and no strong national character had arisen since the days when Nero had taken his 'wife' Sporus about the city displaying him to the populace as he sat, dressed in women's clothes, with full regalia of fashionable paint and powder on his face. Even the soldiers returned from their eastern adventures with outrageous cosmetic fashions, such as gold dust to lighten their hair, and the heavier perfumes which had travelled from the mysterious lands on the way to India.

It was in this period that Cornelius Gallus emerged as a Latin Beerbohm to admit that his lady was improved by rouge . . . or Tyrian vermilion.

The laureate of cosmetics was Ovid, who described the fashion of his day in *The Art of Love,* which was to be reborn with Georgian artifices much later. He followed the general opinion of his time in preferring blondes, and carelessly concludes that no woman need be ugly for all the remedies can be found in pots and lotions. Her eyebrows can be made of fur, a lacklustre cheek can be reddened with rouge, grey hair can be covered with a wig, and patches will emphasize a dull face. Eye shadows could be black or gold, culled from wood ash or saffron.

Martial became angry when men adopted cosmetics to such an extent that they ruined any genuine physical attributes they might have had. The sordid picture of the court of the period suggests dreary creatures, uncertain of sex, who were forced to witness continual tortures and excesses from fear of falling in the imperial esteem, and who plastered white lead and rouge on faces which

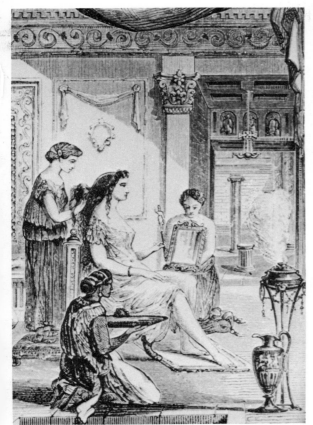
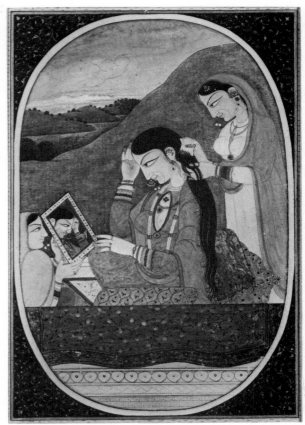

Left: The Toilet of a Roman Matron drawing, nineteenth century
A conception of Roman leisure showing the growing artifice of a woman's toilet.

Right: The Lady and the Mirror 1820. Victoria and Albert Museum, London
The Indian tradition of a scrupulous toilet, here demonstrated by a lady in the nineteenth century.

were no doubt damaged already by ceruse poisoning or by venereal disease. When the Emperor Tiberius finally departed to Capri he was supposed to be blemished by a ruined complexion, and no doubt his followers imitated him in this fashion as in all the others. Martial's refrain is perpetual scorn that his subject could think he did not see beyond the mask. His epigrams, spilling over with venom, attack Polla who dusts her skin to cover the wrinkles, but her dust will not blind the poet; or Aegle who prides herself on her pretty teeth which Martial can see are made out of Indian ivory; or most cruelly, Laetinus whose white hair turns brilliant black, but his mistress knows the truth and will expose him as a senile idiot.

Juvenal was less malicious, and in his writings of about the same period, we can see a more objective view of contemporary fashions. He comments on the high-born prostitute, Messalina, who gilded her nipples when she joined the staff of the brothel; he deplores the women who no longer have to consider their husbands, in this society in which they lead their separate lives, and who loll on sofas all day applying interesting skin packs to their faces, of the type used by the evil Poppaea, Nero's wife.

While the Romans played at orgies and experimented with useless, corrosive cosmetics, the Indians were advancing in their use of cosmetics as allurement. The religious aspect of their painting had ultimately resulted, as in Egypt, with a widespread use of cosmetics in a desire to attract men; for excluding the red mark of the Hindu, paint was used mainly by women. Vatsayana, the compiler of the *Kama Sutra,* probably lived between the first and sixth century AD although it seems almost impossible to date the work accurately. This treatise on love is involved with the religious practices of the time, and it was also intended for a merchant class, in which love of luxury had led the affluent audience to experiment with cosmetics and perfumes, as well as in varieties of sexual pleasure. The wives devoted their time entirely to the master, and they were expected to use cosmetics as an extra weapon in seduction. Apart from studying the *Kama Sutra,* the perfect women should also be skilled in sixty-four extra arts, of which tattooing is number six, and number nine is 'Colouring the teeth, garments, hair, nails and bodies, i.e. staining, dyeing, colouring and painting the same'.

Another skill was the 'art of applying perfumed ointments to the body, and of dressing the hair with unguents and perfumes and braiding it'. There is a chapter dwelling on the daily life of the Indian citizen who would beautify himself after those ritualistic visits to the lavatory and ablutions which were demanded of the Hindu. He would 'wash his teeth, apply a limited quantity of ointments and perfumes to his body, put some ornaments on his person and collyrium on his eyelids and below his eyes, colour his lips with alacktaka, and look at himself in the glass. Having then eaten betel leaves, with other things that give fragrance to the mouth, he should perform his usual business.' The good Hindu also bathed daily, lathered his body every three days, kept his face and head shaved, and removed his body hair every ten days. Sweat must also be wiped from his armpits.

Collyrium was a term for any eyewash or salve; alacktaka was a coloured cosmetic made of lacquer. The bathing rituals were made more easy in later years, when the Mohammedans introduced soap.

Another section in the *Kama Sutra* tells men and women how to make themselves attractive by appearance. The recipe for mascara is written like that of a love potion.

An ointment made of the tabernamontana coronaria, the costus speciosus, or arabicus, and the flacourtia cataphracta, can be used as an ungent of adornment.

If a fine powder is made of the above plants, and applied to the wick of a lamp, which is made to burn with the oil of blue vitriol, the black pigment or lamp black produced therefrom, when applied to the eyelashes, has the effect of making a person look lovely.

The flagrant desire to please which signified an oriental or Asiatic woman was dependent on artifice. In the west at this time, the stern reaction to the decadent Romans had set the culture of cosmetics, like more important arts, back by many centuries. The Indians had no cultural revolution of this type and their sensuality was irrevocably confused with their religious beliefs. When the Europeans encountered these practices of paint, studied seduction, perfume and continual bathing, they were appalled by actions which seemed barbaric, but they were to affect the European culture immeasurably after the crusades. But that was much later; in the time of *Kama Sutra*, the division between the sensual east and the ascetic west seemed, like the thickets of India, impenetrable.

4 Medieval make-up

The fall of Rome was an awesome warning to the rest of the world. It had seemed so unlikely for so long that the great empire might fail; and as the Romans departed from those barren ends of the earth, returning to defend the mother city, it must have appeared as shocking and horrific as if a necessary stream had dried in its bed and never returned.

The Roman armies of occupation have often been depicted as akin to any other occupying army, shown in the New Testament as inhuman automatons of the System, and it is easy to forget how long they stayed in the colonies, for generations of them never saw Rome, and settled in Gaul, Asia or Britain; building houses, breeding children, introducing their own education, mannerisms, attitudes and personal habits. With roads, legality and a unique conception of their own authority, they brought water supplies, clean clothes, cut nails, powdered bodies, washed hair, drainage and perfume to natives who seemed to them as peculiar and outlandish as African pigmies appeared to explorers or Red Indians to white settlers. Those Britons at whom Caesar wondered—coloured with their own pigment, woad—had definitely been impressed by the behaviour of the Romans even if they did not like them. And no tribe, however nationalistic, can remain unapproachable for centuries. The savages who fled across the channel to Ireland, or who hot-footed north from the advancing legions, made a poor choice, for even as serfs the Britons had a better life in the Roman cities than they could have imagined out in the cold swamps, on the bare hills, or running through the impenetrable forests of England. The few mementoes of Roman occupation have become legend rather than report. The opposers of the invaders, confused with earlier and later folk heroes, were so transformed by medieval romances that we can hardly know the truth about the lands occupied by Rome. If we can rely on the scanty evidence of later stories, like those in the *Mabinogian*, we still feel that the princes of Ancient Britain benefited from Roman habits, as even in the most accurate and ancient tale, *The Dream of Maxen LLedys* which is about the Roman occupation, the characters are perfumed, their guests wash, and they wear silk, indubitably in the Latin manner.

After the Romans had washed themselves away, like a tide that would never return, a reaction set in. The water systems, the baths and the chambers where the affluent citizens had perfumed themselves, were overgrown with weeds; by the time a literate record could be made, at about the period of the Domesday Book, the Roman influences have vanished as if they had never been, except in a few preserved but 'lunatic' tales which would be discredited. The victors from the Roman destruction blamed the situation on the Roman character, and all it portrayed to those races which had been observers rather than participants in the imperial glory. Decadence, they said, like so many nonconformist elders, had set in; and in an attempt to halt their own corruption, the ideal personality became one of bravado, with great physical strength and savage attributes, a complete contrast to the Roman ideal man who was clean, intelligent and authoritative, even if he had other traits in common with the barbarians. Through our own concept of heroism, one assumes that the courtiers of Charlemagne, and those Saxons who were close to Leofric, must have bathed, worn clean robes and cut their hair, but if one looks at the primitive homes in which nobles lived, it is only too obvious that under their chain mail the knights were lousy, scrofulous and thick with grime and antique sweat.

As if to emphasize the new age of barbarism, the ornamentation that survived was that of the primitives. The Norsemen, Saxons and Teutons not only coloured themselves with blue dye to alarm their enemies and to act as an amulet against unseen devils, they also tattooed themselves lavishly and crudely. They pierced their ears, and wore thick, heavy, gold jewelry. Their clothes were simple and uninviting, exposing lengths of bare legs and arms. These men were vainglorious, loud in their own praises through sagas and chanted ballads. The women were once more subjugated, animals intended for sex and other heavy duties, and they were expected to present as unattractive faces as their masters. A psychologist might theorize that the vulgar, boisterous world of the barbarian had a current of homosexuality running through it; it is too exclusively the world of men. Vikings expected to sail away westwards for years rather than months, and many women rarely saw their husbands, or those who would have been husbands if they had such formalities as marriage outside the upper classes where marriage was a business arrangement which had to be defined by a contract of possession. There is something too apt about the figure of the page, the boy who runs at his master's stirrup and lies across the foot of his fur-piled bed at night. In later centuries his place would be taken by that dubious figure, the squire; but, regardless of our hindsight, there are no indications that these attendants ever used perfumes or cosmetics.

As Christianity spread, its teaching on personal adornment accorded with the ideas of barbarian rulers. The early Christians were stern about self-indulgence and hardly likely to countenance any suggestion evocative of the wickedness of Rome, particularly a reminder of the corrupt, decorative period. By the sixth century the pleasant relics of Roman rule had been eliminated. The Gauls, for instance, had always been considered a clean, well-groomed race, but this view was swiftly thought old-fashioned. The new élite displayed one alteration during the Dark Ages. The men who had been bearded became clean-shaven as they acquired lands, respect and power. The Normans had been subdued by their comparative affluence in France to discard those signs of the Vikings, the horned helmet, golden beard and tattooed arms. When they came to England they regarded the wild Saxons as anachronisms, for the Norman courtier was smooth-chinned with carefully cut hair. The body of Harold had been recognized after the battle by its distinctive tattoos, including, it was said, 'Edith' over his heart, like any later sailor. This story may have determined the Normans in their aversion to the barbaric habits of the English. They had not tattooed since they had reached Normandy. These tattoo marks were usually tribal symbols, codes for the defeated race, which, strangely, were perpetuated until the present century when some aristocratic Scots were still ceremoniously tattooed with their crests. Obviously, lack of personal adornment became a power symbol, reinforced by the increasingly rigid religious attitudes to cosmetics and even to cleanliness. It is apparent that the early Christian church was thronged with evil-smelling creatures who were proud of peculiarly offensive virtues, such as never washing their feet, changing their clothes, or cutting their nails. At a time when nobody, however eccentric or rich, could be very clean it was difficult but important for the saints to emphasize that they could be even more unpleasant than the general population. It had been ironic that sanitation, baths and perfumes had been included in the general condemnation of the corrupt Romans and it was even more ironic than the reaffirmation of cosmetics came through the church that condemned them.

The first crusade was a revelation to the knights who went on it; not only for its religious significance, but because it carried them out of a life confined to their manor, with an occasional ride to town. Not only did it enable members of a parochial society to break out and visit other countries; it also displayed a form of life that had been forgotten during the Dark Ages.

One can hardly imagine how the eastern Mediterranean must have appealed to some of the northern nobility. It is true that, with typical obstinacy, they described the races they encountered as savage, filthy, avaricious and incredibly cruel—oblivious to their own faults. Yet they encountered habits which ensnared many of them for the rest of their lives, and which impressed them with their artifice. With the more lasting treasures which they conveyed from the eastern lands, they brought perfumes, unguents and cosmetics, along with recipes and notions which their wives seized on with pleasure. Ointments had been medicinal, concocted by witches, who were often accepted members of a small country community. They may have dealt in poisons and love philtres too, but cosmetics had not generally occurred to them. Once the idea of cosmetics had returned to northern Europe, it was only a reasonable time before the same old women could produce a passable imitation of something seen in the east.

Hair dyes were immediately popular with the aristocratic ladies. They changed to blonde or black, but auburn hair had proscribing connotations, being associated with harlotry or witchcraft, part of the folk lore which surrounds a red-haired woman today. The herbal lotions which had been concocted to soothe rashes or skin diseases were now considered face creams which could be used even if there were no disease present, although in the early medieval period there must have been few women who did not need ointments all the time. The crusaders also brought back the idea of removing hair from the body—of women, not themselves, and this was done with a precious piece of pumice, a sharp stone, or with a depilatory cream. In memory of those legendary eastern women, the knights also reintroduced toothpaste as a cosmetic.

These revolutionary ideas were mainly for women; but the baths which had been publicly available in the Near East had appealed to the men, and in some large towns public baths were set up in the main streets and there were even primitive attempts to make the water run, by charging it in through conduits and out through pipes. By the thirteenth century, these public baths were being used fairly regularly by townspeople, and in some areas a recollection of Rome returned, for sweating rooms were added in which eminent citizens would meet to discuss business and local affairs. Some baths admitted women too, with licentious results, for they lay in the same room as the men, separated by a plank table which was covered with sweetmeats. Both sexes were massaged and bathed by naked girls. Although this sounds like a medieval orgy, the baths, were restricted to respectable people, for women with evil reputations and beggars were excluded. These bathing innovations were not encouraged by the church. In France, the Fools' Feasts had been annual excuses for the common people to dress up, play transvestite, paint their faces and lose their inhibitions in orgies which record like evidences of mass hysteria, and they had been banned in 1212. The French churchmen attempted to close the baths too and were largely successful; although the lewder English retained them until 1546. However, they could not levy the same restraints for the aristocracy, and the crusaders continued to have hot baths and steam rooms in the privacy of their increasingly unfortified castles; they even installed primitive sauna baths by wrapping themselves in a garment like a linen bell tent under which they had hot stones. In this ludicrous costume, immobilized by the surrounding stones, they would stand rigidly while their serfs threw water at their steaming white figures. It probably gave the serfs a rare pleasure.

The Jews came in the wake of the crusaders, following the beguiled customers with their offers of spices, dyes, unusual ointments and perfumes. After the thirteenth century a certain number of imported cosmetics were probably available, as well as those innocent ointments which were being made at home from herbs and which were supposedly medicinal.

While some crusaders and their wives were adopting the manners of the Near East, the church became even more restrictive towards the bulk of the population. This was a period in which the peasants were restive and the only authority which the church could ultimately wield was the threat of hell fire. Like the later Puritans, the writers of the period poured wrath on any inclinations to dress attractively, let alone paint the face.

John of Salisbury had seen the way in which women might go during the twelfth century, when he advised men on marriage, exhorting them not to be deceived. A contemporary preacher warned men against women who wore saffron-dyed dresses, a sure sign of whoredom, apart from the sad fact that they looked like yellow frogs, and furthermore painted their faces with 'blaunchet' or wheaten flour to make themselves more alluring. In his tirade he refers to cosmetics as the 'devil's soap'; and mirrors are 'the devil's hiding place'; precursors of later nonconformist attitudes.

By the fourteenth century, religious writers were shaking their heads over the licentious younger generations of women. They had preached modesty as a wife's chief attribute and although cosmetics were so scarce that hardly any account of them survives, the real problem was probably rather less that women painted their faces, than that class systems were breaking down. In the privacy of her home the crusader's wife might have dressed and painted like an eastern courtesan, we do not know, but as the middle classes follow the fashions of their betters, and as the solid goodwife was becoming flighty and given to artifice, one can only suppose that she followed where her superiors had led; for the notion of cosmetics must have come from those social classes which considered themselves above the condemnation of preachers. The religious ideal of the modest woman was evoked by Menagier of Paris:

If you are walking out go with your head turned straight forward, your eyelids low and fixed, and to look straight before you down to the ground at twelve yards, without turning your eyes on man or woman, to the right or to the left,

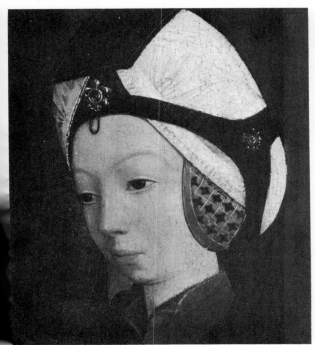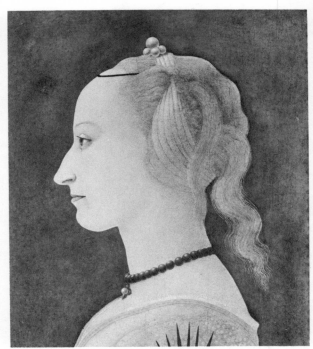

Left Geertgen Tot Sint Jans (*c.* 1460-95) *The Holy Family and their Kindred* Detail. Rijksmuseum, Amsterdam. The medieval face is in this example almost Japanese, with no eyebrows, a small mouth, and downswept eyes.
Right Alesso Baldovinetti (*c.* 1426-99) *Portrait of a Lady in Yellow* National Gallery, London. This late medieval woman could almost have been a figure of the 1920s. Her plucked eyebrows and thin lips reduce the face to the barest details.

or staring upwards or moving your eyes from one place to another, or laughing, or stopping to talk with anyone in the streets.

This demure puss would hardly wear colouring, and in fact, even in the grandest medieval ladies there is little evidence of real colour, for everything was diminuendo. The hair was made pale, and the skin was more pale; by hiding behind the dark walls of the castle, the aristocratic lady retained that whey look which was partly the result of poor diet and partly lack of sunshine. If she did turn brown behind her outdoor veil, she covered her face with a flour powder. This white egg shape reached its apotheosis, if such a plaintive aspect could attain anything so colourful, when the hair was scraped back under an exaggerated headdress and the pallor of the fashionable lady was accentuated by plucking out the eyebrows and the hairline, so that all was smooth, white and without delineation. (See page 27.) The eyes popped like sour gooseberries out of the white face. Those pathetic gothic portraits which we ascribe to the style of painting, were often faithful reproductions of the insipid ladies of the period. Their chief fear was freckles, which would mar the white flatness of the face. What was lost in the complexion was gained in the dress. Wimples, bodices, increasingly ornamented rosaries, and crosses confirmed the aspect of a pious woman but may have made her more exciting to a suitor.

The medieval English court grew more colourful, with harlots like Jane Shore, who certainly painted; homosexuals, who may have; and increasingly complicated fashions in dress, which announced a termination of wars between barons: with the advent of internal peace the individual could go abroad in a velvet coat rather than armour, just as his house could extend horizontally

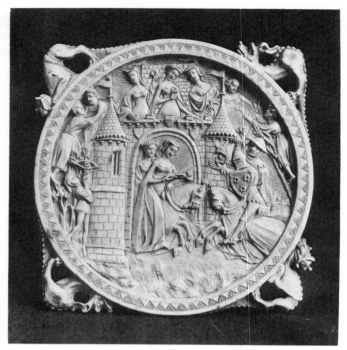

An ivory mirror case, made in France in 1430. Wallace
Collection, London
Although cosmetics had hardly reappeared, mirrors were
becoming more sophisticated.

rather than perpendicularly. National wars continued in spite of the growing
preoccupation with pacific interests such as printing, writing, music and
painting. Softer lines in dress suggested gentler and more courtly attitudes to
other people; although several ghastly internecine wars occurred in various
European countries. In spite of the Wars of the Roses, the power struggles in
Italy and the German states, and the religious unrest in France, the fashionable
people at the end of the Middle Ages displayed remarkable lack of interest in
methods of arming their bodies and houses, and much more enthusiasm for
decoration.

Some of the interest in personal beauty may have been owing to the increased
production of looking glasses, for previously the fashionable ladies had seen
themselves in murky metallic surfaces or relied on other people's reactions to
their appearance. Now they saw themselves for the first time. Some interest
may have been caused by the growth of portraiture during the Renaissance;
for few women had been interested in the ideals of beauty expressed by religious
paintings.

The increasing complications and dissensions in religious belief were also
important in the changing attitudes to make-up; a discreet woman could now
drop somewhere along the way, and follow her inclinations instead of the
teachings of the church. The changing structure of classes had resulted in a
growing merchant class which had no fixed position in feudal society, but
which had money with which to buy new ideas and new commodities. Women
were becoming individuals, and emerging from their slave state, with firm
attitudes to their own adornment. The aristocracy still had the power, the
opportunity and the insouciance to display cosmetics, but the new middle-
class women watched them, and would soon be imitating them.

40

5 The growth of fashion

If the spread of looking glasses and portraiture affected attitudes to cosmetics, it was the personal attributes of women who used make-up that created a demand for it among the upper classes. Although preachers railed against paint and fine clothes throughout the sixteenth century, few members of the vulgar populace actually saw either until the end of the period; for the court ladies passed among them in closed chairs, their beauty hidden behind leather curtains; and even in large cities and the environs of palaces, the faces of aristocratic women were rarely seen. In earlier days they had been hidden by veils, and as fashions in dress changed, they were concealed by vizards or masks. Theoretically intended for modesty, these masks were retained in an immodest age as barriers against the sun, or as weapons in flirtation. The secret dread of most upper-class women was the possession of freckles, which had become as monstrous in the fashionable eye as warts, and were ridiculed ridiculously in a period when scars of disease were so common on the face. During the century, the term was to cover other blemishes, as well as 'sun spots'. Towards the end of the Middle Ages, the use of cosmetics had only been sponsored by notorious women. It is an interesting contradiction which recurs throughout social history that while harlots in high positions were reviled, they were also imitated. Kings' mistresses had no need to hide their shame for they were profiting from it very nicely, and so leaders of fashion were usually those women who would have been outcasts in a more humble or provincial society.

The only other women who could dress and paint as they wished without condemnation were those of such superior birth that they would escape censure from their immediate circle and from the church. Isabeau of Bavaria, for instance, who flourished at the end of the fourteenth century and became the queen of France, was extravagant in attempts to make herself beautiful. Like Cleopatra, she bathed in asses' milk. She must have been one of the earliest slimming fanatics and she would stay for hours in sweating rooms, after which cupping glasses were applied to her body. Her skin lotion was made of boars' brains, crocodile glands and wolves' blood. It was a period when herbal cures, creams and transformation lotions were closely identified with witchcraft, for there is more of magic in the recipes than of common sense. Most of the creams were concocted by awesome old women and had to be applied with incantations.

The European courts of the fifteenth century had many famous male beauties; for kings of both France and England had effeminate traits which were set off by plentiful use of cosmetics. While the majority of women even in high social positions were still hesitant in the use of make-up, Henry III of France had his ear pierced, and went to bed wearing a special mask of flour and whites of eggs, which was removed on the following morning with a sponge dipped in chervil water. Not only was his face painted red and white, but he also plucked his eyebrows and tied his hair up in a false chignon. His attendant young men wore beauty patches in the shapes of flowers and animals. Under his aegis, even wholly masculine men adopted lotions for the skin, rouge and perfumes.

41

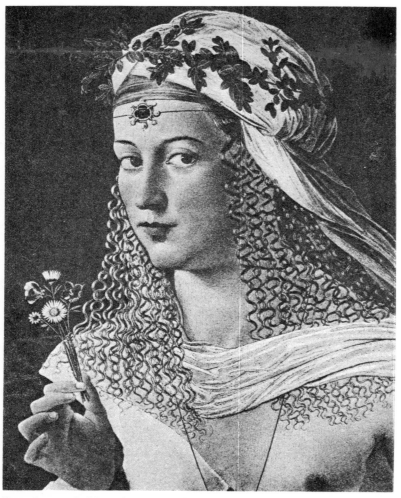

Bartolomeo da Venezia *Lucrezia Borgia* (?) *c.* 1506. Städelsches Kunstinstitut, Frankfurt
The thin, corkscrew ringlets are possibly a wig.

The Middle Ages set the colour for make-up. It seemed wholly natural to later ages that the face should be whitened and the cheeks rouged, emphasizing natural colour beneath; yet studying the colours employed by primitive men, there is no real reason why yellow, blue or black should not be daubed on the face. The red and white design for the face was determined during the Middle Ages as part of the fantasy of the times; for the rose and the lily were the flowers of romantic chivalry, which should be emulated in ladies' faces, and from this time until the late nineteenth century constant evocations of those flowers occur in poems on female beauty. The Renaissance fostered these ideals; and at the same time, the increase in trading facilities brought the tools of make-up to those who could buy them.

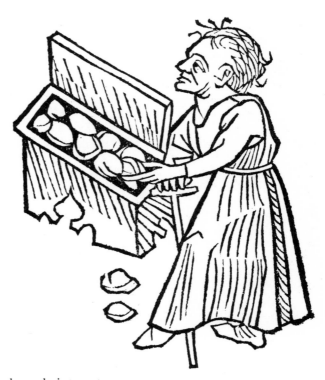

An itinerant pedlar selling herbs and ointments, 1491
This figure suggests that the lower classes were beginning to be apprehensive about their appearance. In some areas the old women would be attacked for witchcraft.

The sixteenth-century beauty looked to Venice to decide her mode of appearance, as a later generation would look to Paris; this position as an arbiter was created not by the Venetian taste, but by ability to supply the goods. The Venetian ceruse was to be considered the best for two hundred years, and its origin gave it a special cachet, women would be deluded into applying ceruse against their own better judgement. This peculiar cosmetic, made of white lead, was to devastate Europe until the nineteenth century. Ceruse was not the only Venetian export, for the rouges of the period also came from Venice, or via its port. Sometimes these were called Indian red, or China, and later, Spanish rouge, but the base, of ochre, was probably common to all of them, and the magic of their names sold them whatever their place of origin might have truly been. In the sixteenth century, all a beauty needed to know was that the best cosmetics came from Venice; and any merchant would also realize that with that fabled tag attached, he could sell anything in a pot.

When the new trade routes to India opened, the Europeans had access to a plethora of new scents, and these became the basic stock in trade of the respectable aristocratic lady bent on conquest, as well as of the prostitute. Even when paint had hardly appeared, sweet smells had been introduced as panaceas for the universal bad ones. In stuffing their noses with strong perfumes, the medieval people hoped to allay the onslaught of plague; in later years, citizens would cover their nostrils with rags soaked in vinegar for the same reason; it was not merely a primitive superstition for there was a desperate chance that air disinfected with such overpowering scent might have been reduced in germs. The French carried 'scent apples' as early as the fourteenth century; these were wooden spheres with holes, filled with a perfumed wax. English women of the middle classes adopted pomanders fifty years later.

Certain scents had long-lasting vogues. The medieval perfume par excellence was of violets which achieved romantic associations as tenuous and pervasive as those of the lily or rose.

Hungary water appeared in 1370, when Charles V of France received some as an ambassadorial gift. It set a fashion which was to persist until the middle of the eighteenth century, with the universal appeal that eau-de-cologne would have later. Composed of a alcohol base with rosemary, cedar and turpentine, it was used lavishly as a rub for the body. Exquisites washed their hair in it as well as their bodies. The most abandoned women soaked sponges and cloths in it and inserted them in their armpits or between their thighs; it probably aided personal hygiene more than water. Soap was still a luxury in the fifteenth century, made up by housewives who might have to resort to rancid animal fat as an ingredient; but the introduction of these cooling waters, and the novel sensation of smelling sweetly, encouraged many of the aristocracy to wash the more intimate parts of their bodies for the first time. A sense of delicacy had been absent from the so-called civilized world for about a thousand years, and the approval of perfumes was the first sign of an appreciation which would ultimately end with sanitation, showers and disinfectants. The most refined and rich aristocracy experimented with air fresheners, perfuming their rooms with 'cyprus oyselet', which was a pomander made of skin which could be puffed into the air, releasing a fine perfumed powder. As windows would hardly open at this period, and rooms were small, dark and close, this innovation must have been a salvation to medieval housewives. There was also revived interest in eau-de-chypre, especially in France. This was similar to the ancient perfume distilled by the Egyptians from Cypriot essences, which had been brought back by the crusaders as an innocuous flower water. The fourteenth-century version was stronger, made of tragacanth, styrax, calamus and labdanum, and the name was altered to 'cyprus' if it found its way into the puffball oysletes. It was also sold in decorative bottles, which were presented as keepsakes in polite society.

The French women were far in front of the English in adaptation to new cosmetics. They had their pomanders, and ceruse distillations while the English were still plucking their front hair and eyebrows, and sponging saffron dye into their poorly shaved scalps. However, they imitated the French swiftly after the rigours of wars and the sparsity of trade had been overcome. As the continental fashions trickled into London, the English churchmen continued to inveigh against feminine vanity which they saw as more than a delusion, a downright danger, for an edict was issued in Elizabeth I's reign declaring that:

Any woman who through the use of false hair, Spanish hair pads, make-up, false hips, steel busks, panniers, high-heeled shoes or other devices, leads a subject of her majesty into marriage, shall be punished with the penalties of witchcraft.

The men who sold the lotions were equally suspect, for they were beginning to approach the lower income groups. In court, the profanity of women was secret, and invisible to the public, but common pedlars were beginning to sell cosmetics, by touting them round provincial fairs. They were still too expensive and daring for a servant girl, and would remain so until the age of multiple stores; but the wives of merchants and the new professional men, would be ensnared by these Tyrian dyes for the cheeks, and blacklead to contour the eyebrows. These shrewd cosmopolitan figures, slipping through the English countryside, could be classed with witches, for they relied largely on superstition to sell their wares, and the habit of producing a universal lotion started in the sixteenth century as fairground buskers realized that no woman would part with her money simply for a face cream. She wanted a magic formula which would also rejuvenate her, eliminate all scars and banish ague at the same time. This determination to have a three-part blessing for the price of one has remained constant in the minds of buskers ever since, incorporated into advertising campaigns and slogans. Sometimes the pedlar went too far and ended in the local jail, denounced as a male witch; but unless his product did actual harm, he probably managed to wheedle his way about the country, for nobody wanted to halt a man who could provide such a precious benefit.

Fifty years later he would be accepted jocularly by most peasant crowds, as Thomas Platter was to find in Avignon in 1598.

Politics, inventions, fashions and arts were all budding in the sixteenth century; by the 1560s there occurred a flowering of every facet of social and artistic life. It was a vigorous time. Nationalism became solidified, for France was uniting and in the titanic wars between continental powers, the beginnings of national characters were forming, based largely upon self-esteem, myth, emulation, and response to desperate situations. The Low Countries, the Italian and German states, Spain and England were all involved in political dog-fights which employed religion as the main weapon. It was necessary for rulers to adopt poses and characters which would enable the people to identify with them; and this exhortation to stand together partially impelled the nobility to mix with the middle classes. Economically, they had to consort with each other anyway; especially in England, where the old social system was breaking up, wrecked by the newly rich merchant classes and the growth of new industries and trades. In the turmoil of the sixteenth century, there was intermarriage between the old nobility and the new bourgeoisie, and the creation of a powerful group of rich men who had done well out of the dissolution of the monasteries and who were prepared to fight to retain what they had won.

Henry VIII was perhaps the first English king with a common touch. His

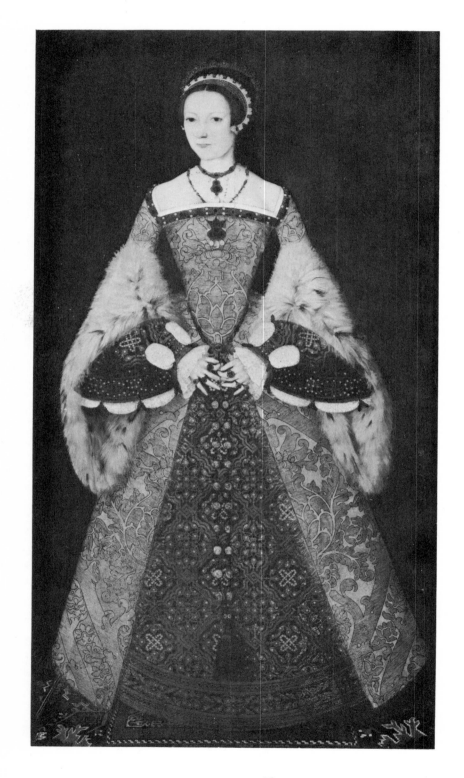

predecessors were shadowy figures to their subjects. Those that stayed at home were invisible except on state occasions, and those who went away, like Richard I, acquired legendary splendour through their absence. Henry VIII made himself a defender of the faith, which aroused acclamation that he was defending an English principle. He moved about the country more than previous monarchs, even if his course tended to run from Hampton Court to Nonsuch. More people had opportunities to see the courtiers, and the merchant classes had a growing sensation that they could not be stopped, and as each man anticipated wealth and grandeur, he sought the means to behave in the fashion of his predecessors, the aristocracy that was becoming extinct. They chose their wives by wealth, but also by appearance. Even Henry VIII had sent careful instructions to his ambassadors when they viewed the newly widowed Queen of Naples for him. They answered his questions with equal care:

Q. Item, specially to mark the favour of her visage, whether she be painted or not . . .
A. As to this article, as far as we can percieve or know, that the said Queen is not painted . . .

Henry was afraid of being caught out by one of those women who, an English moralist was pointing out at the same time, 'whyte theyr face, necke, and pappis with ceruse'.

During the century, the wealth of England increased to the point when its inhabitants might ape the rich Italians in their style of life. It was still a while before they would use cosmetics boldly as part of ritual of everyday life, but the modest woman had vanished as an ideal; perhaps because contact with France had revealed that a rowdy, colourful woman was more pleasurable. Lady Jane Grey, who would have won praise from medieval clerics, was reckoned rather too pale, wan, and gentle in her appearance. Her freckles were considered a great defect, although in this case the term may have been used in its usual general sense of being spots and other blemishes. However, small and humble though she might appear, there was no doubt in onlookers' minds that she was remarkably clever, even in using those few attractions she might have had, for a visiting Genoese thought her 'graceful and well made', if small, and 'when she smiled she showed her teeth which are white and sharp'. She was also acute enough to wear 'chopines' on state occasions, which were high-platformed shoes to increase her height. But, alas, the passing of that pale demure girl marked the end of a romantic view of women. She was perhaps the last of the quiet women who did not raise their heads too high, but like many of them, she displayed self-control and stubborn determination when they were necessary; her relative, who fostered cosmetic arts as a tabby fosters her glossy coat, was as different as fire from water. Elizabeth was a prototype of the twentieth century woman.

Master John *Lady Jane Grey* c. 1545 National Portrait Gallery, London

6 The acceptance of cosmetics

Cosmetics came into general use during the reign of Elizabeth I, and as the acceptance of them was owing to her, that livid face should be studied before those of her courtiers.

In her youth, vanquishing foolish boys, playing mouse to her sister, Elizabeth was supposed to be an attractive girl. Her qualities were so far removed from the romantic medieval conceptions of beauty, that one feels that even in these she is more comparable with twentieth-century women than with those living between her and them. Her splendour came almost wholly from her personality. Even as a girl, with a prim face, reddish hair and heavy-lidded eyes, there was no doubt of the force of character behind the face which attracted men, and then repelled them. Stories about her sex life are so confused and unreliable that one can only imagine it. In her youth she wished for flirting, loving and sexual contact, providing it made no indentation on her own vigorous personality. In spite of her reputed moanings about being a barren stock, the thought of Elizabeth with children is ludicrous; she was a career woman. She enjoyed admiration even if she was astute enough to realize it was not always sincere. She was vain, as many women are who hover between extreme ugliness and distinction. Her handsome face would have been too harsh without make-up. She presented a mask which was enamelled into a nothing face. At a period when portrait painters were beginning to show something of the spirit of their sitters, she displays nothing except a composed visor. As she grew older, cosmetics became currency among the aristocracy, but Elizabeth amazed the most sophisticated ambassadors by the exaggeration of her artifice. 'Her hair was of a light colour never made by nature', and as her jawline fell in from lack of teeth and her hair disappeared, the queen became even more extravagant in her use of cosmetics, leading the fashion of her time.

Few elegant ladies desisted. They dyed their hair, plucked their eyebrows, covered their exposed breasts with white plaster and painted their faces. The revolution was in the foundation of their beauty rather than the addition of colour, although that was startling enough. Lotions, potions, ointments and creams were churned out by alchemical confidence tricksters or in the still rooms and bedchambers of country houses. 'Water to make women beautiful forever' has a charming ingenuity, but the composition of most of these preparations was not innocent. A young raven was taken from its nest, fed on hard-boiled eggs for forty days, then killed. The flesh was distilled with myrtle leaves, and the noxious result should have transformed the buyer. Two 'brand name' lotions appeared in the sixteenth century which were to survive for the next two hundred years. One was Soliman, or Soliman's Water, obviously a derivation from Solomon, who was still a magical name in necromancy. It was supposed to eliminate all spots, freckles and warts, and its chief ingredient was sublimate of mercury which polished off the outer layer of skin and corroded the flesh beneath. The girl's teeth fell out even more rapidly than was usual at this date, her gums receded, and by the age of thirty the devotee of miracle lotions would be a rotting wreck.

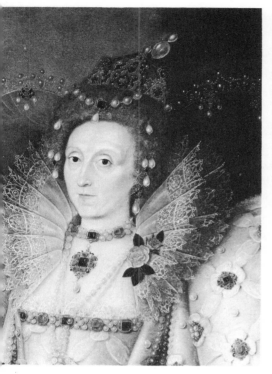 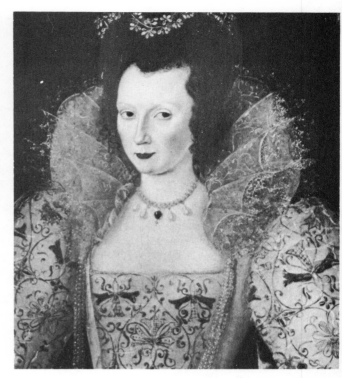

Left Marcus Gheeraerts the Younger *Queen Elizabeth I* c. 1592 National Portrait Gallery, London

Right: Elizabethan Lady late sixteenth century. Bodleian Library, Oxford
This portrait is unusual in its depiction of cosmetics.

The other longstanding remedy for faults in the complexion was less debilitating, but of little use; Tristram's Water became a houshold standby, distilled in country kitchens for centuries out of oil of bay, rhubarb, spices and wine which were steeped for a month. Maturity was of great consequence in the legends of beauty preparations, and as most of the blemishes appeared during the summer, the familiar stench of soaking herbs and fat-filled wine vinegar must have been indelibly associated with fairer faces. In those days, when a freckle could cover a variety of skin problems, incantations existed which might banish them by moonlight in a fusion of elder leaves, sap from birch trees or powdered brimstone mixed with turpentine, which was left on the blemish until morning, and wiped off with the fresh butter drawn of that morning's milk. The lily face was to remain the most desirable until the middle of the twentieth century and face whiteners were devised which incorporated lemon juice and egg white—one of the most pleasant remedies. Eczema conditions could be cured with whole eggs, dock roots and brimstone flowers simmered together for three days. This condition, and other similar scurvy ailments, were termed the 'white Morphew' and would only be remedied, in time, by changes in diet.

Upon this unsure complexion base an enamel was set, the usual main ingredient being egg white, which dried out to a fine glaze like that seen on china. The famous ceruse, compounded of white lead and vinegar, was also used for the best effects. The ladies who could not afford this cosmetic saved their skins unintentionally by making do with sulphur and borax. These poor innocents would contrive to make their lips red with a mixture of hard-boiled egg white, cochineal and gum arabic. Those ladies they envied would use the permanent red of fucus which was the cosmetic term for red mercuric sulphide. When he explored Guiana, Sir Walter Raleigh was to compare this dye with that of the natives which was superior, made of 'divers berries, that die a most perfect crimson and Carnation. And for painting, all France, Italy or the East Indies, yeild none such: For the more the skyn is washed, the fayrer the cullour appeareth . . . '

Some unfortunates blushed involuntarily, and in a time when a red face would suggest a choleric temperament, many fashionable ladies and gentlemen attempted to subdue their natural ruddiness. One man slept with double linen socks on his feet which were filled with dry powdered Bay salt. He washed them out each morning, possibly believing that the salt had drawn the evil humours out of his body through his feet, and that washing would kill them.

Few middle-class people cared about their teeth. They were certainly well rid of them when sore gums and rotten molars ruined the peace of everybody over twenty-five. The courtesan had always been aware of the distress of stinking breath, and as the upper classes became more sensitive to smell, they could only emulate her methods of controlling it. The queen was so concerned with smell that all about her courted favour by smelling sweetly. It was usual to connect scent with sweet taste and early mouth washes were made of spiced wine. When it became obvious that teeth must be cleaned to achieve true sweetness, most families concocted tooth-powders of honey and sugar; or crushed bones and fruit peel. Burnt alum and ground rosemary was made into a more astringent paste. They were applied with tooth cloths of coarse linen, and after rubbing industriously with these, the mouth was washed out with wine or a sugary water. Unpleasant stains on the teeth were removed with pumice powder mixed with pulverized coral, brick, and other abrasives, which removed the enamel as well as the stain. Courtiers had elaborate tooth-picks of precious metals decorated with jewels. Humbler people used iron or wooden toothpicks. If all these measures failed, many Elizabethans resorted to the more familiar trick of keeping their mouths closed.

When none of the cosmetics succeeded in beautifying her, a woman had the recourse of hiding her face behind a mask, so that only her intimates saw her. However, her bosom would be displayed if she were unmarried, which ensured that the queen had opportunities to exhibit hers until she died in her seventieth year. Her breasts were whitened with the everlasting ceruse, which many of her subjects imitated, delineating their veins with blue liner. The other inescapable exhibit was hair. The passion for blondes was well established in England at this time, and many women dyed their hair, perhaps with this recipe: 'Take the rine or scrapings of Rubarbe, and stiepe it in white wine or in cleare lie'. A more extreme, but no doubt certain, method, was to dip the hair in oil of vitriol, turmeric or alum water. Obstinate brunettes powdered their hair with yellow powder or gold dust. In the early years of Elizabeth's reign, the hair was often concealed under a snood or wimple, but as the queen grew older her styles of hairdressing became more ornate and macabre, and so did her subjects'; with vast edifices of curls which were rigidly beaten into shape with irons, then lacquered with a strong smelling pomade. If there was enough hair, it was mounted on a pad, but if it had grown scanty with old age or too virulent dyes, it was enhanced with false hair. Lacking the prey which had been available to the Romans, the rich Elizabethans had to find their false hair where they could, and pay dearly for it, usually buying children's hair, or sending into the country for it. The gallants of Elizabeth's court vied with women in experimenting with skin lotions, dyes and cosmetics. To later readers, there seems some incongruity between the portrait of the complete Elizabethan . . . soldier, explorer, wit, athlete and poet . . . and the portrait of the same man, enamelled with as much fervour as a fashion-conscious woman. They promenaded before the queen, perfumed in a hitherto unimaginable way and outdoing each other with varieties of beards, hose, hats and ruffs. Not only did they practise forms of posture in the corridors about the court, they would also have been seen ogling themselves in a corner where they could see by the light of a window. Their mirrors would have been made of glass in rare cases, but more often of polished steel, and they were carried in the hat brim. They were acutely complexion-conscious, occasionally using masks to protect their faces from the sun. It was customary to dye one's beard auburn as a compliment to Gloriana, to wear a large earring in one ear, to carry perfumed gloves, and to grow one lock to hang down, with a ribbon knotting it at the shoulder.

Their chief pleasure was in perfume, for the Elizabethans had a large number of new smells to content them, and their hypersensitive queen. From the east came civet, ambergris and musk, and those were added to recipes which had already made English toilet waters famous on the continent. An amateur alchemist, Ralph Rabbards, sent a note to Elizabeth offering his services as perfumer and promising her 'waters of purest substance from odors flowers, fruites and herbes wholesomest, perfitest and of greates vertue are first distilled by desensory, dpeured and rectified, clere as crystall, with his onlie proper virtue, tatse and odor contyuing for many years'. As in so many delightful country perfumes of the period, he relied on 'jilly-flower and pinckes'. The scents were not in the liquid form known today, but appeared as a powder, paste or thick gelatinous mixture, as there was no known method of diluting them or of extracting essential oils. The natural perfumes from flowers, musk, or ambergris were mixed with sugar and simmered for several hours. The result must have been overpowering. The Italians showed their skill in perfumery as they did in cosmetics, for a leading chef in the world of perfumes was Master Alexis of Piedmont, whose damask water, a favourite among his customers, was made from musk, ambergris, sugar, benjamin, storax, calamus and aloes wood beaten to a fine powder 'and put together in a little perfume pan, pour in as much Rose water as will be two fingers high and make under it a small fire that it may not boil, and when the water is consumed you shall pour in another and continue this doing a certain number of days'. The paste form of perfumes made it expedient to use them in pomanders and pouncet boxes which nobles carried about in their hands. The originals had been oranges stuck with cloves, or else filled with a cloth or sponge soaked in aromatic herbs and vinegar, but a society accustomed to jewelled toothpicks could hardly countenance such a simple method of keeping the plague away. Pomanders became increasingly ornate.

Hair was perfumed and so were clothes. Gloves were the most usual form of perfuming, especially as leather retained the smell; but stockings were scented, as well as belts and necklaces. Bags of lavender were laid to rest with sheets which had already been washed in rosewater. Cushions filled with dried petals lay about the rooms, the walls were even washed with rosewater, especially at court, for Elizabeth had it made by her maids and also imported it in bulk.

This ostentatious allegiance to paint, perfumes and conceits disturbed the growing numbers of Puritans. They reproved those women who patted about the court in high heels, thrusting up their painted breasts with tight corsets, flaunting their grotesque red curls, and rolling their kohl-lined eyes which had been illuminated by belladonna. John Knox had poured the wrath of God down upon Mary, Queen of Scots as a papist murderess, but one feels he was more incensed by her baths of wine and by that strange skin, whiter than her snow-white veil, which stilled observers, and made men fall ridiculously in love with her. Elizabeth's face had none of that charm, and few of her satellites could approach it either, but they became a cynosure for fanatical preachers. Philip Stubbs, a puritan cleric, railed at the women of his time, damning 'whosoever do colour their faces or their hair with any unnatural colour, they begin to prognosticate of what colour they shall be in hell'.

Apart from the outcry on going to God with a face which was not one's own, there was a more comprehensible fear that the cosmetics might do harm. Chemistry was advanced enough for scientific writers to suggest that white lead was corrosive although they had no notion of the internal problems it might cause. However, the world ran on make-up and as it was the rage no woman of consequence would be deterred. By the end of the sixteenth century a hint of satire had crept in, and the woman painted with a false mask was introduced as a figure of fun in contemporary plays; but gently, for the most artificial of them all was still in command, and as Elizabeth grew older she became more concerned with her vanishing looks. She outlawed looking glasses from her household and sometimes sat in the dark, perhaps because the injuries of injudicious painting were beginning to show, or else the result of strong chemicals had made her fearful of exposing her damaged skin. She was made up by maids who saw her as a figure of fun. According to Ben Jonson she 'never saw herself after she became old in a true glass; they painted her, and sometymes would vermilion her nose'.

Foreigners admired the Englishwomen, finding them easy to talk to, open in their friendship and accustomed to walking about the streets and visiting the taverns without specious modesty. They bought their cosmetics in the streets from hucksters, or went boldly into the fashionable shops where milliners (or men dealing in Milan wares) displayed the most exquisite linens, gloves and ribbons, all perfumed to please the English taste.

The French became as bold as the Englishwomen under the tutelage of Catherine de Medici, whose attitudes to fashion were almost as exaggerated

There was often a narrow demarcation line between cosmetics and medicine; in the early seventeenth century quacks sold both. This pedlar is selling the Theriak, a cure-all made, it was claimed, from snake's flesh.

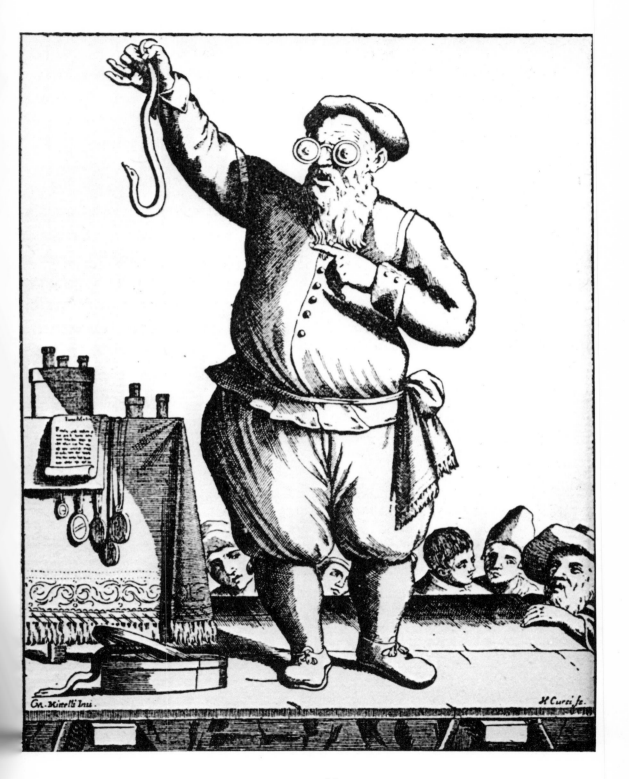

as those of Elizabeth. The men of Paris used cosmetics, beauty patches and powder on their hair as ably as the London gallants. The Germans were still dour, living in a puritan society where women retained something of the modesty of the medieval wife. When men from northern Europe did travel abroad they were overwhelmed with the strangeness and richness of the more licentious lands. Thomas Platter went to Montpellier from Basle at the end of the sixteenth century to study medicine. At the age of twenty, his record is simple, observant and concerned largely with those scenes which differed from his customary surroundings. In Spain he wrote:

Spanish women are very fond of their toilette and love nothing so much as to beautify themselves. The hem of their dress contains a wooden hoop to hold it out, and to allow them to walk with greater dignity. They also generally wear pantaloons under their skirts. Their slippers are of a prodigious height. The fashion is to put on an outrageous amount of powder and paint on the face, the throat and the hands. The colour is supplied in little pots, one of which I sent to Basle. From this comes a saying that alludes to this painting and these shoes: Who has a Spanish Wife has four: one tall and one short, one beautiful and one plain.

Thomas Platter also described the vendor of cosmetics, half rogue, half doctor, a character who has played a role in so many historical novels that he is almost submerged by imaginative incarnations. Shakespeare describes him as Autolycus, the clown-pedlar in *The Winter's Tale*. From Platter we have a lengthy account of a man who brought lotions and pastes from the east, or more probably from his own stewpan, to sell to gullible ladies at country fairs. Zani and his company were also actors. They made their sales talk into a show in which the character of Doctor Pantalon criticized the magic ointments which Zani ably upheld. Finally the price came down:

. . . to five crowns, then two, then one, then to ten stübers, to five, to two . . . and he called out yet more strongly to the people to pass their money to him in their handkerchiefs and even promised an extra box for those who were first. The handkerchiefs came at once, and in great numbers, to be returned to their owners with the precious unguent. In some instances, the actresses included little notes to give the time and place of a rendezvous.

After having sold several hundred boxes in this way, Zani urged the tardy to hasten, for the last few boxes were in his hands, and he would not have any more afterwards: the morrow would be given over to quite different things. In fact, the next day, at the same hour, the play being done, he exhibited dentifrice powders in perfumed envelopes, pastes to kill warts, or cure aching eyeballs or toothache; Venetian soap; scented waters etc. Zani sold them for a stüber after the same little act as before.

7 The milkmaid
and the merchant's wife

All her teeth were made in Blackfriars, both her eyebrows in the Strand and her hair in Silver Street . . . she goes to bed with some twenty boxes.

Ben Jonson commented in *The Silent Woman* on a common joke which was amazingly new, for the people about whom he wrote are hardly of high social status; his characters are merchants, and all the classifications below them, including thieves, servants, artisans and layabouts. The woman who was over-cosmeticized, a walking prop for artifice, had descended in the social scale. He was however writing about London, which had grown so much in the years of Elizabeth that many poets and playwrights had idyllic dreams about the countryside which was close to them but which they rarely had time to visit, unless they had some pastime or excuse, like Isaak Walton. The romantic poets at the beginning of the seventeenth century also had visions of a girl who was untainted by the veneer of London and who was typified by Sir Thomas Overbury as one of his characters, the milkmaid,

. . . a country wench which is so far from making herself beautiful by art that one look of her's is able to put all the face physick out of countenance . . . her breath is all her own, and scents all year long of June, like a new mown hay cock.

Overbury preached the fashionable jargon but his own affairs were bound up with the fatal Countess of Essex who finally was purported to have conspired to kill him, having her poisons made up for her by the alchemical lady who was also supposed to supply her with cosmetic lotions. The court was given over to cosmetics when James I came south with his tall blonde Danish wife, Anne. The enthusiasm for all types of extravagant living was a world away from the climate of thought in Edinburgh; London ladies wore cosmetics to court so continually that a woman who appeared without them was an original.

The Countess of Bedford . . . who should have gone to the spa but for lack of money, shows herself again at Court, though in her sickness she had in a manner vowed never to come there. . . . Marry, she is somewhat reformed in her attire, and forbears painting, which they say makes her look strangely, among so many vizards, which with their frizzled powedered hair makes them all look alike so that you can scant know one from another at first view.

The country did succeed where the town failed in one aspect. Those dangerous recipes incorporating chemicals were losing ground with some perceptive women, though they hardly replaced their compounds of vitriol with more useful unguents. Dog urine, pulverized minerals and infused flowers were ruthlessly blended to form household recipes for beauty. The time of the milkmaid had come, in that her dairy could be robbed of the best cream for some new complexion milk.

The seeming growth of household recipes is probably illusory, arising from the fact that women were writing down their secrets and passing them on to their daughters. It was still the moneyed classes, stirring away in manor house kitchens, who attempted to right their wrongs with cosmetics. Their behaviour was noted by their maids however and many country remedies of the eighteenth century had their origin in a home where the more humble women watched their mistresses, unable to write down the instructions, and then repeated a garbled version in their own kitchens. Necromancy was to creep into reasonable recipes by this back door; for the creams which were concocted had to be implemented by magic if they were to work for people who still saw fairies.

There is sometimes a strange illogical plausibility about the home-made remedies. Chapped lips could be cured, for instance by detaching the sweat from behind the ears and rubbing it on the mouth, which would grease the cracks. Limestone was boiled in water and when it had been cooked for a lengthy time it was mixed with soap and rubbed on to warts, and the secession of the wens was less due to the soap and the spells than to the action of the lime.

Some remedies might induce internal upsets but few could have been as insensately cruel as that practised by William Butler for a man cursed with a red face. John Aubrey tells the tale in *Brief Lives*; as Butler died in 1618, this anecdote must date from the early part of the century:

A Gent. with a red ugly pumpled face came to hime for a cure. Said the Dr. I must hang you. So presently he had a device made ready to hang him from a Beame in the roome, and when he was e'en almost dead, he cutt the veins that fed these pumples and lett out the black ugley Bloud, and cured him.

In addition to writing recipes in notebooks which were to be kept for the family, a new interest had arisen in printed books concerned with food and medicine. The new professional classes, which were becoming increasingly important, relied on books to communicate with each other. Books had been limited in the sixteenth century to religious works and a few publications which already had a proved market before they came out. In the seventeenth century medical books, memoirs and the first few works of fiction were to become popular. In 1597 *Gerard's Herbal* was published, but it became known in the 1633 edition which had been revised by Thomas Johnson. Most of the considerations are medical, but as a poor complexion was, rightly, interpreted as a medical problem, there are tantalizing glimpses in the *Herbal* of the brewing and gathering necessary to produce a clear skin. Cucumbers could be used as an inward remedy eaten as a potage with oatmeal and mutton; or alternatively used as an ointment. A dish of cucumbers taken:

. . . for the space of three weeks together without intermission, doth perfectly cure all manner of sauce flegme and copper faces, red and shining fierie noses (as red as Red roses) with pimples, pumples, rubies and such like . . .

Provided alwaies that during the time of curing you doe use to wash or bathe the face with this liqor following.

Take a pint of strong white vinegre, pouder of the roots of Ireos or Orrice three dragmes, searced or bloted into most fine dust. Brimmestone in fine pouder halfe an ounce, Camphire two dragmes, stamped with two blanched Almonds, foure Oke apples cut thorow the middle, and the juyce of foure limons; put them all together in a strong double glasse, shake them together very strongly, setting the same in the Sunne for the space of ten daies: with which let the face be washed and bathed daily, suffering it to drie of it selfe without wiping it away. This doth not onely helpe fierie faces, but also taketh away lentils, spots, morphew, Sun-burne and all other deformities of the face.

He also observes:

The distilled water of the floure of Rosemary being drunke at morning and evening first and last, taketh away the stench of the mouth and breath, and maketh it very sweet, if there be added thereto, to steep or infuse for certain dates, a few Cloves, Mace, Cinnamon, and a little Annise seed.

In spite of these romantic cure-alls and the literary interest in dew-washed maidens, at the court of James I the plaster was laid on as thickly as ever. The court entertainments were usually masques, elaborately engineered vehicles for the queen's pleasure, at one time designed by Ben Jonson and Inigo Jones. The atmosphere was completely at odds with the age which was to follow it and which already existed in public imagination. Like a dinosaur the Jacobean court life lumbered heavily across the London stage, with courtiers dressed in heavy padded garments, stiff, old-fashioned farthingales and thick make-up through which they peered dimly at the outside world. The faces of James and his consort, stodgy and old before their time, are at complete variance with the light clear faces of Charles I and his family as depicted by Van Dyck. These portraits show them dressed in loose, elaborate but graceful clothes, and seemingly remarkably lacking in make-up. In spite of the king's own inability to relax, the court was less urban than it had been for several reigns, Henrietta presumably wore make-up but it is not obtrusive, and the portraits and letters of the time suggest that make-up was worn but with more discretion than it had been for fifty years.

The court picture was at variance again with the outside world. Its informality and casual grace was alien to the burgher class who were still involved with the decorations which had typified the upper classes previously. It is difficult to pursue a god for years and then discover he has another face. The merchants' wives ignored the relaxation at court; the queen was described as brown-skinned and monkey-faced, so she must have spared the ceruse, and in fact she asked the court physician, Sir Theodore Mayerne, to prepare an alternative. But the lawyers' wives and the rich women who were beginning to move to suburban houses, still wished to wear the trappings that had always denoted rank and wealth. It was this middle class, agog for new delights and contrivances, that Shadwell was assessing when he made Harty address Clarinda and Miranda in *The Virtuoso*, offering them:

. . . choice good Gloves, Amber, Orangery, Genoa, Romane, Frangipand, Neroly, Tuberose, Jessamine, and Marshal, and all manner of Tires for the Head, Lock, Toms, Frouzes and so fourth; and all manner of Washes, Almond Water, and Mercury-water for the Complexion; the best Peter and Spanish paper that ever came over; the best Pomatums of Europe, but one rare one made of Lamb's Caul and May-Dew . . . Also all manner of Confections of Mercury and Hogs-Bones, to preserve present and restore Lost Beauty . . .

The list of perfume includes many names which were to remain popular during the century. Neroli was made for the wife of the Duke of Neroli;

Frangipani was a new scent to the English and French but it had been a favourite in Italy which was revived by the descendant of the Frangipani family who was a marshal of Louis XIII's army and wore gloves scented with his ancestor's perfume. Marshall was probably derived from Poudre à la Maréchale d'Aumont, which was powder sold in sachets and which was added to a cream or paste to form a scent in conjunction with other essences.

Women's complexions were at this time concealed completely by the mask. As these became part of their daily wear they were developed into two types. The traditional mask was oval, made of leather, velvet or some other black fabric stiffened with canvas. It was held in place by a bead gripped between the teeth. Half masks succeeded but did not replace them. They stretched over the upper part of the face and were tied behind with laces or ribbons. By the 1630s they had been accepted by the middle classes as well as by the aristocracy, and well-heeled merchants' wives customarily wore them when they were shopping, or walking in the open spaces which were common in London. The mask extended its duty by night for complexions were protected by similar veils which were placed over a creamed face and drawn tightly to press out the wrinkles. Theoretically these variations on the net were of fine fabric such as silk, thin cotton or linen, but many women must have utilized those day masks which had grown too shabby for the street, and especially as more sophisticated ones were lined with silk or fine kid, and many men must have been alarmed by the head on their pillows, disguised with black leather.

> Here be fine night masks,
> Plaster'd well within,
> To supple wrinkles and to smooth the skin.

wrote Michael Drayton in *The Muses' Elysium,* and for good measure he also mentioned the gloves which were used to keep hands white:

> . . . searcloth gloves doth show
> To make their hands as white as swan or snow.

This was in 1630. The passion for cosmetics had reached stronger proportions in Paris where the nuns were said to pass about the streets with their hair fashionably curled and powdered. Powder was being used in advance of its time for the apotheosis of puffballs and flour was to come over a hundred years later. However, in the 1630s the working-class French women were covering their heads with flour or turning it auburn with rotten oak powder. The richer women utilized their hair powder in a paste which they smoothed over their heads. Its perfume was appropriate to the colouring of the wearer. Cyprus oil was universal but blondes favoured iris scent, and dark women used violet.

In France the men were considered advanced in foppery, but the English gentry of the period were not far behind them; neither nation cared for bathing at this period although the English were already castigating the southern Europeans for their filthy habits. The Grand Tour was to become the finishing

Opposite Engraving after Hollar, 1643
The mask only disappeared from fashion when the simplified styles of the 'classical' period became popular at the end of the eighteenth century. Until then it was a partial disguise and therefore a weapon in flirtation, and a protection against the weather when creams were uncertain allies.

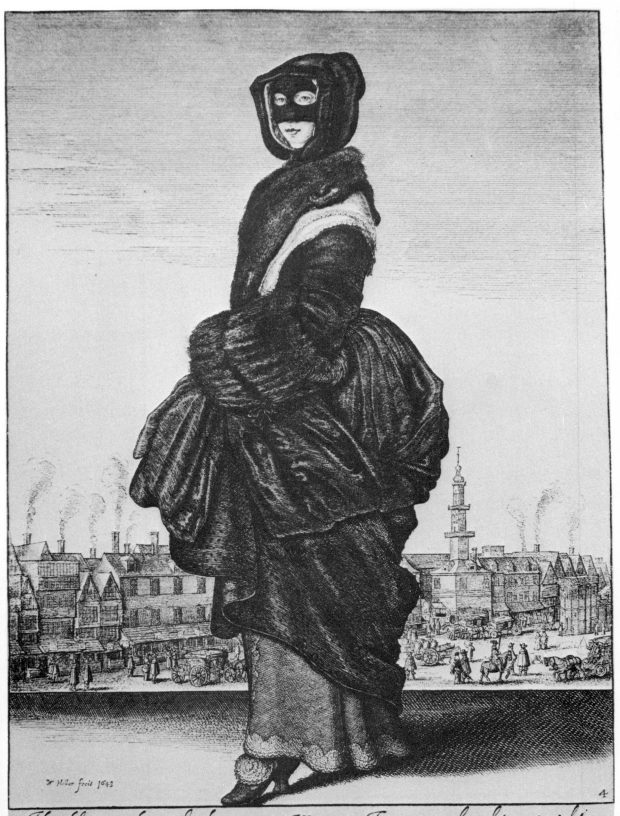

W Hollar fecit 1643

4

The cold, not cruelty makes her weare   **Winter**   For a smoother skinn at night,
In Winter, furrs: and Wild beasts haire   Embraceth her with more delight.

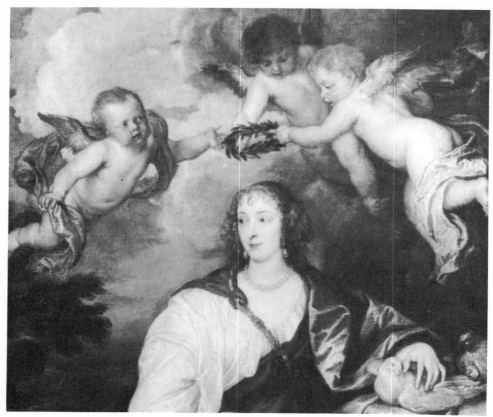

Van Dyck *Venetia Stanley, Lady Digby c.* 1633. Detail. Private collection

school of Englishmen during the next century but even in the early seventeenth century Italy was often the subject of a year out of society for the upper-class English, particularly those of aesthetic humours. Charles I's only adventure was when he went to Spain to woo a princess, but his friends were of more cosmopolitan minds. Arundel, his adviser on paintings, was a suave dilettante who patronized Hollar and Harvey, and encouraged the king to buy Italian paintings. Another friend was Endymion Porter who married a Spanish lady; it was a closed circle round the king which had the attributes of an exclusive club, the admittance fee being an interest in painting, architecture, music and masques. The members were not necessarily powerful, rich or noble, in fact the company of plain gentlemen might even have been a relief to the king, who accepted any opportunity to avoid political reality. His wife, petulant, francophile and light-headed, was also pleased to have charming men about her who could flatter her with a grace which she considered continental. One of this group was Sir Kenelm Digby who was not only a great original, but who devoted much of his time to writing down common knowledge of the time which would otherwise have been forgotten. *The Queen's Closet Open'd* was one of the first collections of household simples. Digby created a scandal when he married Venetia Stanley in 1625. Although she was accepted as one of the beauties of the age, she was an acknowledged courtesan and had previously had an affair with the Earl of Dorset. Digby seems to have had no qualms about her history, (she was of the same social class as himself) and in spite of her retinue of followers, for Dorset was not her only lover, Digby insisted that he would make her virtuous. He was so self-possessed that he sued the earl for the annuity he had settled on Venetia as payment for her services, and won the case. It is interesting to see what this paragon of beauty looked like, in the words of that shockingly blunt man, John Aubrey:

She had a most lovely and sweete turn'd face, delicate darke-brown haire. She had a perfect healthy constitution; strong; good skin; well-proportioned; much enclining to a Bona Roba (near altogether). Her face, a short ovall; darke-browne eie-browes about which much sweetness, as also in the opening of her eie-lidds. The colour of her cheekes was just that of the Damaske rose, which is neither too hotte nor too pale. She was of a just stature, not very tall.

This suggests more of the pretty milkmaid than of the bedizened ladies of whom Jonson wrote. But even she was apt to overdo her skin treatments, or else her husband became reckless in his attitude towards her beauty. He was jealous for her and she led a sad strict life according to her female friends who passed the news on until it reached Aubrey, who repeated the story that she had died of an overdose of a concoction given to her by her alchemist husband to preserve her beauty.

She might have done better with Gervase Markham's advice. He was another of the same type as Kenelm Digby, noting down the recipes and remedies of the period for publication. His bath would not actually injure a woman's beauty and might even sustain her:

Take rosemary, Feverfew, Orgaine, Pellitory of the wall, Fennell, Mallowes, Violet leaves and nettles, boil all these together, and when it is well sodden, put to it two or three gallons of milk, then let the party stand or sit in it for an hour or two, the bath reaching up to the stomach and when they come out, they must go to bed and sweat, and beware taking of cold.

Auburn dye had become démodé with the death of the old queen and golden hair was all the rage again. Rhubarb was still the sovereign base for the colour, mixed with white wine, although honey and gum arabic was a popular recipe.

In addition to ceruse, a whitener for the face was made of powdered pig-bone. Rouge had become cheap, even the servants could buy plenty for a penny. It was a different conception from the beauty of Venetia Digby and the results would hardly please the gentlemen of the court, but city dwellers had become accustomed to bright colours on ladies' faces.

All this painting and powdering brought a spate of satire too. John Donne could make a teasing conundrum out of the proposition *That Women Ought to Paint*: 'What thou lovest in her face is colour, and painting gives that, but thou hatest it, not because it is, but because thou knowest it.' The man who supplied the art was rising in the world. There were no luxurious beauty parlours, but there was Dr Plasterface, as seen by John Marston in *The Malcontent*, the forerunner of many similar characters in the business of cosmetics.

By this curde, he is the most exquisite in forging of veins, sprightning of eyes, dying of hair, sleeking of skinnes, blushing of cheeks, surphleing of breasts, blanching and bleaching of teeth, that ever made an old lady gracious by candlelight.

8 Restoration beauties

Cosmetics should have been outlawed from the period of Parliamentary rule. Reading the accounts of the strict régimes of those days, when paintings were burnt because they showed nude bodies, and the façade of St Paul's was allowed to tumble down because it represented a decorative attitude to worship, it is amazing that cosmetics survived. In a world where it always seemed to be winter, with monochrome figures moving across a darkened landscape, the women are represented as forbiddingly plain, with no touch of lace, or curls. In America, this lachrymose spirit was even more enduring and girls who wore innocent ornaments were handed before a judge. Yet patches were used, as they had been more or less since the reign of Edward IV. Their numbers had increased during the last half century, and in 1653 an English writer says, 'Our ladies here have lately entertained a vaine custome of spotting their faces, out of an affectation, of a mole, to set off their beauty, such as Venus had'. In May 1654, John Evelyn noticed that 'Women do began to paint themselves, formerly a most ignominious thing and used onlie by prostitutes', which suggests a poor memory. Country girls may have been treating their skins for that could surely not have been considered a trap set by Satan; and in 1652 *Culpeper's Herbal* was published, telling interested readers that burned walnut ash would turn their hair yellow, or that blackberry leaves boiled in water would dye it black. Culpeper adds gratuitous information about French dames using the pimpernel to make an infusion which smoothed rough skins.

While John Evelyn abhorred the indecorous Englishwoman who painted her face, he seems to have found the Venetian ladies wholly charming as they sat in their windows in the sun, drying their hair by spreading it out over the brim of a crownless hat, through which they had pulled their long 'crisped' locks. With naked arms showing through false sleeves of tiffany, and a yellow veil over the rest of their bodies, they must have appeared more mythical than real, which probably made them a suitable sight for an academic visitor.

The Restoration brought an inevitable, and eagerly expected, reaction. A court which had been sated with France, but which had grown accustomed to the extravagances of the Parisian life, would hardly bear the dull faces of modest Englishwomen, and the women of a generation which was hardly removed from that which had encouraged the happy milkmaid of the 1630s, gratefully began to colour their faces, bleach their hair and whiten their breasts.

The middle classes aped the court, as they had done in the past; but now the court was not so exclusive. The king and his mistresses could be seen walking in the park, and there seems to have been no barrier to keep them from the palace, where Charles's friends, at least one child, and his mistresses, attempted to remain equable in their crowded lodgings.

Pepys strolled about Whitehall, noticing every change in habit and fashion. It was he who commented that Cromwell's daughter joined in the race to follow the latest craze: 'She put on her vizard and so kept it on all the play; which of late is become a great fashion among the ladies, and which hides their whole face.' (June 12th, 1663)

These masks were still retained, mainly out of modesty among the middle classes, but at court they were tools of the game, used for flirtations. In 1660, Mrs Pepys put on her first black patch. It was probably a spot of black taffeta; or it may have been red and cut out of Spanish leather. They were usually placed near the mouth. Patches would enlarge to ridiculous sizes and patterns, but initially they were simply 'mouches', or love spots, which, said the king's mistress, Lady Castlemaine, 'All fashionable ladies should wear all the time, unless they were in mourning'. Her decree was probably superfluous, for women were already blotching their faces with larger and more complicated patches, and in 1667 the Duchess of Newcastle made the patch look ludicrous by appearing in 'a black velvet cap, her curls about her ears and lavish patches on her mouth, because of the pimples'.

Patches appeared on the customary skin of white ceruse. The best ceruse still came from Venice, for the English was inferior, in that it had less white lead. It was mixed on a palette, with water or egg white, and applied to the skin with a damp cloth. The scarlet which was laid over this whitewash was sometimes Indian lake or cochineal. It was a shellac obtained by melting and refining the resin from a tree of the acacia family. It was worked until it achieved the correct lacquer consistency.

Few women needed to mix their own colours, for rouge was more commonly applied from Spanish paper, Spanish felt or Spanish wool, which was impregnated with a dye which could be rubbed on to dampened cheeks. The consequent red and white face was irritating some observers even then. De Grammont, the laconic observer of English ladies at the court, noticed that the famous Mrs Wetenhall, who had been praised as a rare beauty, looked like a doll.

Samuel Butler, whose epic political satire *Hubidras* appeared during the reign of Charles II, commented at the time on the accepted beauty:

> Her mouth compar'd t'an Oysters, with
> A row of Pearl in't stead of Teeth
> Others make posies of her cheeks;
> Where red and whitest Colours mix;
> In which the Lilly and the Rose,
> For Indian Lake and Ceruse goes,
> The Sun and Moon by her bright Eyes
> Eclips'd and darken'd in the Skies
> Are but black patches that she wears,
> Cut into Suns and Moons and Stars.

The memorable women of the Restoration were rarely good, if sometimes kind. The courtesan had come into her own; from Lucy Walter, that pseudo-wife of the young king's exile, who was described as brown-skinned, to Barbara Palmer, later Lady Cleveland, who was a paragon of red and white sophistication. The Restoration face, plump, slack-lipped and double-chinned, seemed destined for marshmallow colours, indeed it is difficult to imagine it without powder and the ubiquitous patch.

In his memoirs, ghosted by Anthony Hamilton, the Count de Grammont described the beauties of the court in a less agreeable manner than Sir Peter Lely, who painted the harem for the walls of Hampton Court. Mrs Hyde was to become the wife of James, Duke of York, the king's brother who would later

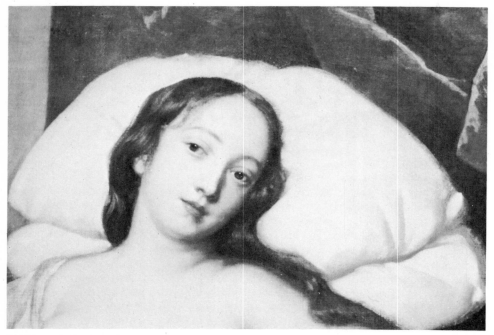

Sir Peter Lely *Nell Gwynn* (?) *c.* 1670. Detail. Denys Bower Collection, Chiddingstone Castle, Kent
The face of the Restoration beauty was delicately coloured and voluptuous. This is alternately supposed to be Barbara Villiers and Nell Gwynn.

be James II. 'She was of middle size, had a skin of dazzling whiteness, and a foot surprisingly beautiful, even in England: long custom had given such a languishing tenderness to her looks that she never opened her eyes but like a Chinese; and, when she ogled, one would have thought she was doing something else.' The most engaging young beauty was Miss Hamilton, 'she was the original after which all the young ladies copied in their taste and air of dress. Her forehead was open, white and smooth; her hair was well set, and fell with ease into that natural order which it is so difficult to imitate. Her complexion was possessed of a certain freshness, not to be equalled by borrowed colours . . .' She is an absolute contrast to the unfortunate Miss Blague, who was, says the unkind Hamilton, 'another species of ridicule: her shape was neither good nor bad: her countenance bore the appearance of the greatest insipidity, and her complexion was the same all over; with two little hollow eyes, adorned with white eyelashes, as long as one's finger.' Miss Blague definitely had no appreciation of cosmetics.

If fair complexions were outlawed, it was in celebration of those brown-skinned beauties who came after Lucy Walter. Hamilton describes Miss Bagot as having 'beautiful and regular features, and that sort of brown complexion which, when in perfection, is so particularly fascinating, and more especially in England where it is so uncommon. There was an involuntary blush almost continually in her cheek, without having anything to blush for . . . .'

64

It was unusual for a woman to have nothing to blush for in a society where infidelity was applauded and rewarded, and most women seemed chaste if they had only one lover. Marriage was the key to promiscuity, for when there was no longer a virginity to lose, many young wives adopted the manners of the court and received their lovers when their husbands had gone to business. The comedies of Wycherly mirror an age and an appetite which was quite astounding. If he exaggerated, other and less sparkling writers repeated the basic rules of the game.

The bravest sparks . . . like caul cats in March run mewing and yawling at the doors of young Gentlewomen; and if any of these have but a small matter of more than ordinary beauty, (which perhaps is gotten by the help of a damm'd bewitched pot of paint) she is immediately adored like a Saint upon an altar.

So said Mrs Aphra Behn in her serious and caustic book, *The Pleasures of Marriage*.

These lascivious she-cats entertained, for the first time, men above stairs. The dressing room was not yet the parlour of the eighteenth century, but already intimate friends could expect to meet there. These congregations began with some respect, as young wives gathered to congratulate a new mother, then casually entertained each other in their bedrooms; and finally they allowed everybody in. The audience was not always engaged in admiration and attention. Although nobody was as pitiless as Swift would be on the subject, the items on a dressing table could be as carefully enumerated by Mary Evelyn:

> Of toilet plate, Gilt and Emboss'd
> And several other things of Cost,
> The Table Mirror, one Glue Pot,
> One for Pomatum, and what not?
> Of Washes, unguents and Cosmeticks.
> A Pair of Silver Candlesticks;
> Snuffers and Snuff-dish, Boxes more
> For Powders, Patches, Waters store . . .'

Like the ancient Egyptians, where the rich fashionable family could not carry their wealth in their face, they placed it in the boxes which held those faces. Expensive toilet sets were made to special order for the famous beauties of the day; some were given as wedding presents, like that presented to his wife by Sir Walter Calverley in 1716, which was made of silver gilt, and very costly. Small boxes and toilet articles were often made of gold and silver. They were not as flamboyant as the spirit of the age might suggest, for though portraits might have become great classical conversation pieces, and cosmetics had more of the stage than of the street, the tweezers, bowls and boxes were of baroque silver gilt, and are surprisingly refined. This may have echoed the growing refinement of their owners. In spite of the loose morals and the bawdy language the bourgeoisie were becoming conscious of the crudities of everyday life, like dirt. The plague was an abrupt reminder of primitive dangers in a civilized world: and many intelligent, if profligate, men and women considered cleanliness as essential, rather than peculiar. Invaluable Hamilton recounts that the ladies of the court were accustomed to bathe, for one of his long anecdotes of jealousy and machination takes place in a bathing place. From the story we learn that a lady, tired and heated by riding, asked leave to change her linen in another's room. Miss Hobart, the hostess, exclaims with pleasure at her guest's clean habits, and adds to the charming Miss Temple that she compares well with another lady of the court, Miss Jennings, whose ears must have burned holes in her mask-strings at the conversation. 'I am enchanted' (says the viperous Miss Hobart) 'with your particular attention to cleanliness: how greatly you differ in this, as in many other things, from that silly creature Jennings! Have you remarked how all our court fops admire her for her brilliant complexion, which perhaps, after all, is not wholly her own; . . . What stories I have heard of her sluttishness! No cat ever dreaded water so much as she does: fie upon her! Never to wash for her own comfort, and only to attend to those parts which must necessarily be seen, such as the neck and hands.' Upon which, Miss Hobart aided her friend in undressing, and led her to the bathing closet where both of them sat on a couch to continue their interesting conversation.

Hamilton's picture of the bath, glass-screened and curtained with Indian silk, is a curious one, reminiscent of a Turkish idyll, and perhaps owing something to one, for after the emissaries of Turkey had appeared at court, fashion flitted after them, and eastern manners were adopted, as well as strange westernized modes of Turkish dress, which resolved as baggy pantaloons and silk turbans. The men of the time had every pleasure, not only could they wear cosmetics with impunity, but they seized every opportunity to assert their masculinity. It is an interesting consideration that fashions in sex seem to follow the pattern in power as well as they do in politics or dress; for at the lively heterosexual court of Charles II there were no overt homosexuals. Instead, most of the men boasted of their conquests, not in the anxious manner of the unsure, but with a nonchalance which suggested that sex was fun.

The opposite was true of part of the court of Louis XIV, where Monsieur, the king's brother, had favourites, and was notoriously ornate in his dress and cosmetics. Not that this would signify a homosexual—far from it, the beaux of Restoration England had proved that; but as most memoir writers of the period mention Monsieur's paint, they were merely adding a final proof of his extravagant oddity.

Most men exhibited their love of adornment with wigs and perfumed waters. The wig may have been introduced to polite seventeenth-century society by Louis XIII, at a period when long hair was the prerogative of the well born, no doubt to indicate that they had time to curl it and no hard work to sully it. When the king grew thin, then bald, a wig was brought in to supplement his own hair, and from this an elaboration resulted in an edifice, a curled and periwigged monstrosity.

Charles II was prematurely grizzled, and although admirers may feel that his grim face was better offset by grey, he substituted a wig for his own hair, and approved a fashion which was to last until the end of the eighteenth century. The wig was not a burden, although it seems so to present day observers; it was indeed a liberation. For the first time since the Normans, the gentle-born could cut their hair. Strangely, no adherent of Charles II ever considered that he was similar to his father's enemies, as he cropped his hair short to the scalp, or even shaved it off. Mrs Pepys was ahead of her husband in the fashion, buying a peruque in 1662. A year later he considered a wig, but that meant two . . . an expensive commitment. At the end of the year he actually bought one, deciding that he would no longer have to worry about keeping his hair clean. Learning that Duke of York was going to buy one, Pepys essayed his own, with great trepidation, for his hair had to go. He was hooked. Two years later he grew his hair once more, but returned to his wig again. It was too convenient, and on hot days a gentleman might remove it and wear a night-cap or a silk handkerchief in his own home.

Men might also wear scented waters. The smell of their ornamental kerchiefs languishing on a summer wind as one walked in Hyde Park, must have been one of the delights and follies of the age. The Elizabethan idea of scented gloves had persisted, along with pomanders and puffballs to clear the air in the room. The powders which were sprayed out were called 'pulvills'. Hungary water was still the most popular perfume for the home and it would be made in the still rooms of country houses. Urban dwellers imported it from Amsterdam. Civet, ambergris and musk formed the basic scents; there were two types of chypre. 'Red' chypre was a rose smell compounded of damask roses, sandal-wood, aloes, cloves and the familiar trio: musk, ambergris and civet. Chypre was also the familiar name for a dry perfume made of benzoin, coriander, cataminth, storax and calamus root. It would be used for perfuming clothes and closets, and also to puff into gloves. These home-made scents might be any type the maker desired, and the young ladies of the time must have employed hours in the summer, adding and subtracting oil of lavender, marshall, civet and jessamine butter. This last perfume came into the country, as an oil, from Amsterdam, and it was often used in making perfumed gloves.

At the end of Charles II's reign, many perfumes were available in shops, and fashionable characters would gather to smell over the newest imports at shops like the one kept by Mr Charles Lillie at the corner of Beaufort Buildings in the Strand. Previously the main fashion importers had congregated at Cheapside or Holborn, but as the fire and the plague had finally guaranteed the westward progress of the town, shops opened in the new areas of St James's which had no association with past trades . . . in the preceding century a perfumer would have built his business around a basic employment, such as drapery, or a chirurgeon's practice, or a barber's shop, and there would not have been enough custom for him to specialize in one of the luxury trades, dependent on imported goods and the vagaries of fashion. After the destruction of the city, and the old city traditions and trades, a shop could be exclusive and committed to superficialities. Perfumers also sold chicken-skin gloves which fine ladies wore on their hands at night, probably filled with cream, or a concoction of almond paste, ox gall and egg yolk. Plumpers would be sold under the counter, for no woman would admit to wearing them. They were small balls of cork which filled out the hollows left in cheeks after the teeth had gone, 'much used by old Court Countesses' observed John Evelyn in the *Fop's Dictionary* of 1690. Belladonna was sold, to add lustre to eyes, but the mascara which accompanied them was not the eye cosmetic we know today, it was smeared on the upper lids, but it was red, like the henna used in the east.

It was safer to buy a hair dye from a shop than to attempt to concoct one's own, which could have disastrous results; as Lord Ormonde would have remembered from the days when he had spied for the king in exile, secretly entering England from France and dyeing his hair to match the ragged dress he affected. His hair turned bright and varied colours and created a story that Ormonde told with pleasure in the palmy days of the Restoration. Black hair was considered attractive, but gaining it was another problem . . . a 'gum dye' of walnut peelings, myrtle leaves and sage was one solution; another recipe created nitric acid by advising one to dissolve a groat in aqua fortis, and then to wash the hair with the liquid. This approval of brunettes was peculiar to the Restoration court, and so were new theories about beauty which would not reappear until the twentieth century. The court beauties seem dull, fat wenches to us, but they had a charming spite and a false sympathy which is almost endearing. Stories of Nell Gwynn are common, but they do underline the new comprehension of the period which was to be deluged by the dull tedium of the next three reigns.

Charles II was personally responsible for many of the better aspects of his court; the lack of class consciousness arose from the arrival of humble girls who became royal mistresses. The easy mixing between actors and courtiers suggests the beginning of a fashionable egalitarian spirit. In terms of beauty, the period was notable in accepting as attractive women who would not have fulfilled the requirements of later fashions. De Grammont's partiality for brown-skinned girls suggests this quirk. He also mentioned for the first time that a man with a strong and damaged face might be more attractive than one with perfect features, saying of Lord Arlington, 'He had a scar across his nose, which was covered by a long patch, or rather by a small plaster, in form of a lozenge . . . Scars on the face commonly give a man a fierce and martial air, which sets him off to advantage.'

The Restoration playwrights pinned down the fop, the butterfly who was to be even more in evidence at the beginning of the next century, and who was typified by Monsieur, the king's brother, in France. The difference lies in character, for the beaux of Congreve, Etherege and Vanbrugh have a soft centre as well as a soft shell, and Monsieur was all steel under his effeminate exterior. He got what he wanted. He was disliked and feared by the court of Louis XIV, where men could not easily dismiss a man who was supposed to have murdered his wife, Charles II's sister, Henrietta Maria.

The court of the newly established Versailles was more formal and more dangerous than that of England, and the cosmetics were suitably sophisticated. In 1675 Ninon de Lenclos, the mistress of the late king, said that she owed her beauty at the age of sixty to cosmetics, but she was preaching to the converted; every silly whim and fashion was vaunted, put down, and torn to shreds by the women of the court. Their face creams were famous, and exported to England. The faces of the most noted belles were doll-like, aspiring to that of Lady Wishfort in *The Way of the World,* who had 'cracks discernible in the white Vernish', if she smiled. The beauty parlour originated in France, in Paris at this time, with shady establishments next door to large households, where jaded gentlemen and even ladies, might go to have baths and massage. The women might have depilatory baths, especially if they had failed with the famous household recipes for removing hair: fifty-two egg shells beaten and distilled to paste; or powdered cat dung mixed with wine vinegar.

These parlours were often brothels in disguise, or they would let out rooms to couples making assignments; in one of them the king met his future valet, la Vienne, who was making a handsome living at his job of providing girls to amuse the clients, compounding virility pills or procuring abortions. When he became the first gentleman's gentleman, he had to shave the king every two days and bathe him with wine and cold cream. His task was hardly arduous however, for Louis instituted the *levée* and accordingly relegated duties to every high-ranking member of the court; and so that none might be excluded, a wide variety of small tasks were defined, which had to be performed every morning. Monsieur's special job was to pass the royal napkin, which was a hot cloth, used to wipe the royal hands. They could not be dipped in water, it would be too abrasive. His rooms and all the state apartments, were perfumed continually by pages who had to ensure that the air was always sweet with scents of rosewater, sweet marjoram or mallow. Many women spent great sums in having new perfumes created for them, certain that they might attract the king by their odour; it was customary to use a different smell each day, and Madame de Pompadour would bring this passion to its peak in the reign of the next king by making a perfume 'bank' which cost one million francs.

This later extravagance made even the Sun King's excesses seem normal, if not reasonable. In a world where the court was divorced from the outside world in its own village of Versailles, there could be no contact with the middle classes, who could not see, and imitate, the exquisites. Cosmetics were in a vacuum, never departing from the confines of the court. Thick enamel was criticized but not discarded. Madame de Sévigné noticed that even a Hugeonot girl was painted. Yet virtue was triumphant, when Louis XIV passed over the enamelled beauties for Louise de la Vallière who was too religious to paint. Addison commented on the French shame when the ladies of Versailles met a comparatively simple English woman, the Duchess of Manchester:

When the proud ladies of France who cover their pale cheeks with artificial rouge, saw this beautiful foreigner shining like a goddess although only wearing what Nature had endowed her with, their look betrayed their confusion, and a natural blush crept into their cheeks.

9 The rigid Society

In England the ox-eyed Caroline beauties disappeared, in the form of ungainly Lely and Kneller canvases, to dusty eighteenth-century attics. Their languor was outmoded, and so were those low-swathed gowns which had always seemed on the point of absolute departure. Rigidity was to replace the voluptuous style. There is little attractive in the austere profile of the William and Mary figure. Even the domestic arts reflected the mode of dress: plain-faced brick houses were surrounded by formal gardens with clipped hedges in the Dutch manner; and in every elegant reception room, waiting as company for lonely visitors stood monstrous dull figures, cut from wood and painted to resemble odious two-dimensional humans who attended intimate conversations with a sly and satisfied air of abstraction.

These stiff dummy populaces represent the age, for although the coffee-house customers continued their salacious easy conversations, the fashionable people were bound by habits as rigorous as their dress. Consider the woman of 1700. She wears a head-dress which has all the clumsy ineloquence of a folded fan; and under it her body is defined in a cast-iron mould; narrowed skirt, tight bodice and crimpled lace front make her into a doll herself. By the turn of the century, the 'face' has arrived, a face which is as definite and unalterable as the dial of a clock, without the attraction of mobility which signifies a clock face. For the last sign in the female face of the century would be the passage of time. Young and old . . . the plasterwork was the same. After 1700, the satirists could jeer and the young girls sigh, but the age of painted ladies was anybody's guess. Matthew Prior wrote:

Stiff in Brocade and pinch'd in Stays,   Paint, Patches, Jewels laid aside,
Her patches, Paint and Jewels on;   At night Astronomers agree,
All Day let Envy view her Face: The Evening has the Day bely'd
And Phyllis is but Twenty-one.   And Phyllis is some Forty-three.

Make-up continued to increase in popularity. Cosmetics had been available, but now there was a new class to wear them. As transport was organized, local shops could keep secret supplies of foreign cosmetics, and out-of-town misses could paint themselves with as much equanimity as court ladies; and the growth of the cities signalled the arrival of a new moneyed class.

There had been a society of opportunists since the Restoration. It had caused great political heart-searchings, for the morals of the old Royalist aristocracy had been useful to the Stuart crown. These ancient gentry had been diehards for old ways, for stubborn loyalties which had been shaken by the events at the end of the seventeenth century; and their attitudes would now be relegated to the attics along with the family portraits. There was an altered pattern in town life. The squires and their wives were of the past, and although they still existed and might ocasionally struggle to Whitehall to prove it, their way of life was dodo-dead.

It was fashion which mattered in Augustan London, and as critics pointed out, if you were not fashionable you were nowhere. The rakes of the Restoration seem to have been playing delightful games compared with the society which succeeded them. The new people were not aristocracy in the ancient sense, but they were rich. They had two traits which would have been unacceptable in their class before; they were primarily fashionable town dwellers, and they did not work for their living. Divorced from provincial problems, they had no duties to perform.

They behaved in the manner which was expected of them. There was little room for real eccentricity in the new aristocrat. In plays of the period the 'loony', the bait, and the dullard is the man who tends his acres in the country, or who sits in his library alone. This society was gregarious. Cosmetics were worn as a matter of course, and no lady could venture out without her plastered face; the milkmaid had departed and the new aim was sophistication.

Previous customs and designs were submitted to the straitjacket of the age. It is typified by Congreve, who translated Ovid's *Art of Love* into stanzas which read like the advice column of a women's magazine:

> I need not warn you of too pow'rful smells
> Which sometimes Health, or Kindly Heat expels.
> Nor, from your tender Legs to pluck with Care
> The casual Growth of all unseemly Hair . . .
> Yet, let me warn you, that, thro' no Neglect,
> You let your Teeth disclose the least Defect.
> You know the use of white to make you fair,
> And how, with red, lost Colour to repair . . .
> Marrow of stag, nor your Pomatums try,
> Nor clean your furry teeth, when Men are by . . .

Ovid was also plundered by the period for recipes for complexion creams. His *Art of Beauty*, translated (also by Congreve) for the dressing rooms of Augustan beauties, suggests more sensible concoctions than their contemporary beauticians:

> Vetches and beaten Barley let them take,
> And with the Whites of Eggs a mixture make;
> Then dry the precious Paste with Sun and Wind,
> And into Powder very gently grind.
> Get Hartshorn next, (but let it be the first
> That Creature sheds), and beat it well to dust.
> Six pound in all: Then mix and fist 'em well,
> And think the while how fond Narcissus fell . . .

In the same translation concoctions are recited containing Flower de Lis, Lupin seeds and the inevitable Ceruse, this time appearing as a remedy for freckles; which would certainly conceal them. A mixture of rose leaves, frankincense, malt and a mysterious Sal Armoniack would create a 'Rosy Blush', while the more impatient beauties could daub their cheeks with a mixture of poppy petals and water.

One of the new modes, which must have been one of the most difficult to emulate, was to have pleasant teeth. Previous generations had accepted blackened stumps as a fatality of age, which occurred while most of them were hardly past their first youth. Dentists were still the chirurgeon barbers, whose status was so low that a man of refinement, let alone intelligence, would never consider it a profession. In fear of pain, most people, in any stratum of society, avoided tooth pulling, but by the early eighteenth century teeth were considered a possible attraction and experiments were made to replace carious and lost teeth with a false set.

There had been previous attempts to thread wood or bone on to wire and insert them into the mouth. They had been clumsy as well as painful. In the early years of the century denture plates were still wooden platforms into which ivory shapes were fixed, bound on to spiral springs. In 1728 a French dentist, Pierre Fronchard, made false teeth from gold plate with teeth of jewellers' enamel. These imitations could not appear too white or regular however, for nobody had teeth of that regularity and tint. It is not surprising that a genuinely foppish courtier, like John, Lord Harvey, should appear with something approximating to the real article: 'slim, exquisitely dressed, painted, and with the finest set of Egyptian pebble teeth'.

Although Harvey, that celebrated 'butterfly, that thing of silk' as Pope described him, had notoriously depraved tastes, he was probably not unique in using paint. Men wished to have the uniform beauty of the period too, and town air would hardly affect a false complexion, for so many of the fops of the early eighteenth century appear to have hardly stirred out of doors. Shopping, the great recreation for fashionable society in later periods, had hardly progressed to comfort. The noisome streets and ill-lit shops were not enticing. Most rich men ordered their goods and their tailors, hairdressers and perfumers waited upon them at home.

The characteristics of Queen Anne's reign sometimes seem to be a superfluity of time and a minimum of imagination. This was the first time Society had a capital 'S'. Probably there had never been such a consciousness of class difference. Servants were kept in their place and there were assuming their own airs and graces, the world of fashion hardly noticed the poverty in the city; they were removed, as never before, by the possession of wealth.

As the merchant classes gained more wealth and a section of society did not have to do any work for its living, hours could be spent at the dressing table by both men and women. The growth of leisure among the rich town-dwellers created a whole new concourse of tradesmen to cater for them. Perfumers were now distinct from chemists, hairdressers were soon to establish an ascendancy unknown in any other age except our own, and as the rich grew richer, and time appeared to be less and less valuable, artifice supplanted artifice until the face was obliterated by what went on to it.

The ultimate fashion was the patch. In the reign of Queen Anne the tiny black shapes reached their apotheosis. A French commentator, Hubert Misson, describing the English in 1698 said, 'In England, the young, old, handsome, ugly, are all bepatched till they are bed-rid. I have often counted fifteen Patches or more, upon the Swarthy, wrinkled phiz of a Hag three-score and ten and upwards . . .'

They were originally intended to cover blemishes, and therefore they had some necessity in a world persecuted and marked by smallpox, but in an artificial society they became a game, a symbol of sentiment, as superficial and unnecessary as the Language of the Fan.

In London they were political. Whigs wore them on the right cheek, Tories on the left. But this economy in patching could hardly have been endearing to a society which fixed them, in increasing complication, over the face and bosom like so many cooks sticking sixpences into a pudding. The shapes became more involved and ludicrous, those simple crescents and spots which had satisfied the Restoration ladies were quite supplanted by coaches with six horses (which must have caused some problems of space), stars and birds. In France, patches were even more ingenious. The Marquis de Zenobia went to a party wearing sixteen patches, one of them a tree holding two lovebirds.

At the court of Louis XV the patch achieved a loquacity unparalleled in England. The corner of the eye indicated passion, the centre of the cheek was gay, the nose was obviously saucy. A patch on the upper lip suggested kisses, the forehead meant majestic. Worn on a dimple it was playful: and a murderess, if only in the cause of love and intrigue, wore her patches on her breast.

Complexion milks were sold under brand names for the first time. Until the end of the seventeenth century most women had made their own herbal creams, relying on traditional recipes or experimenting with flower extracts and more violent ingredients. Dung, minced veal, and goat hair were still allayed with lemon juice, milk or cucumber water. The complexion did not improve, and so the beauty would lay even more colour on her face. There were some cure-all lotions which acquired a legendary reputation as advertising and report were accelerated. The sovereign remedies, which were to beauty what the Philosopher's Stone or the Elixir of Life had become in the world of chemistry, were continually reappearing under different guises. They not only healed the skin, they supposedly healed the body as well, imitating the well-known chant of Zani, the actor, long before in Avignon.

The most notable lotion was the Chemical Wash which had already appeared in the previous century. Newspapers and imaginative producers made it the most miraculous ointment in the history of beauty treatments:

for making the skin so delicately soft and smooth, as not to be parallelled by either wash, Powder, Cosmetick etc. being indeed a real beautifier of the Skin, by taking off all Deformaties, as Tetters, Ringworms, Morphew, Sun-Burn, Scurf, Pimples, Pits or Redness of the Small-Pox, keeping it of a lasting and extreme Whiteness; they soon alter red or rough hands, and are admiral in shaving the Head: which not only gives a more Exquisite sharpness to the Razor, but so comforts the Brain and Nerves, as to prevent catching cold, and are of a grateful and pleasing scent.

This advertisement suggests that the beauties realized that their skin cures and cosmetics could do more harm than good, but they persevered in using them.

There was no relief from the scorbutic countenance. Complexions continued to be scarred, sallow and spotted. They could only be covered. The most immediate remedy was the mask. Decent women had worn masks out of doors before, they became even more important in Georgian London. They had lost their utility as a protection against cold and prying eyes, and had become the weapon of a coquette. It was less usual for men to wear masks although Venetians used them, as we see in paintings by Longhi.

Masks were made of black silk or velvet, stiffened with fine leather or buckram. The more common type was the half-shape which circled the eyes and tied behind the head with ribbons. The full face mask was still used on the continent but had less popularity in England. It was too formal. The beaded

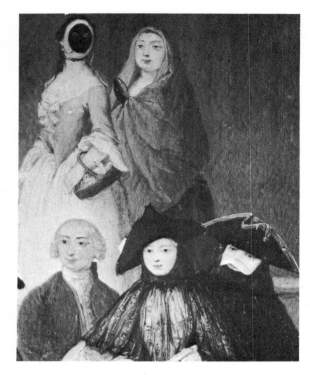

Pietro Longhi *The Masked Visitors at a Menagerie c.* 1750. Detail. National Gallery, London
Longhi painted cruelly satirical views of Venetian life in which masks became more sinister, concealing the lusting face of an old man; or covering a woman's features with an uncanny oval shape.

fastening restricted speech and movement and could have caused unpleasant accidents. But the masks for the upper face had the charm of a masquerade. As the pleasure gardens were opened, and offered opportunities for affairs, clandestine meetings and a pretence of democratic congregation, the mask became a uniform, to be worn for seduction.

Their attraction may explain the relative unimportance of eye make-up. The Georgians had to exert their skill on colouring lower down in the face.

This colouring, the clearly defined red and white, was to remain constant until the end of the century. The white was the customary ceruse but it had spread to a larger section of society than ever before. The rouge was usually called 'Spanish red' and it arrived in an impregnated pad of hair, like today's Brillo pad, and producing much the same results.

The all-pervading colour was used by both sexes. In 1735, fashionable magazines referred to a beau as 'red'ning his lips and painting his nauseous phiz' and at about the same time there were allusions to a Guards' officer who wore patches like a coquette.

As we have seen in advertisements, the Georgians were aware of the dangers of indiscriminate make-up but persisted in using it. The most noted victim of cosmetics was the beautiful Maria Gunning. (See page 101.)

This daughter of an Irish squireen who assailed London society with her sister Elizabeth, had a season of triumph and retired to marry the Earl of Coventry. He disapproved of cosmetics, to the point of scrubbing her face with a napkin before guests at a dinner in honour of their marriage. After this unfortunate beginning, the new Lady Coventry appeared at court a few days later, and either pique or indifference had made her paint her face with the white lead again, to a becoming but obviously artificial pallor, which caused comment in the magazines. In spite of public criticism the two sisters were still the darlings of the crowd, although Foote, the famous actor-comedian of the times said that 'They were just married in time, for another month would have brought them from goddesses down to the level of mere women.'

For two years, Maria played the part of a countess with unexpected decorum, although her vanity was considered ludicrous by everybody except her admirers. She didn't look her best or dance in assemblies and a cruel friend reported that the Gunnings were not happy as mortals after a spell as society beauties. In 1756 she lost her decorum, and caused a minor scandal by receiving a lover in her box at the opera. After being the wonder of all the gay world, pretty Maria Gunning had become the object of its spite when she appeared as Lady Coventry. Maria's vanity was the subject of satire. Her strings of lovers, as well bred as racehorses, trotted after her as she moved from town to country and back again; and over all, her pale face became paler, accentuated by reckless if skilful applications of ceruse.

As the snow dissolved in 1760 she was imitating it. Her doctors reproved her for persisting in her increasingly hectic social life. She had an obsession with her own beauty which had made her one of the sights of her time. As Lady Coventry she could hardly permit herself to dismiss the shade of the beautiful Miss Gunning. In January she went to the hot wells at Bristol, which, not surprisingly, gave her little relief; and so she returned to town to attend the trial of Earl Ferrers. The visit was a social necessity to her, for all the wits and gossips of the court assembled to hear sentence of death passed on the criminal and to watch him hang, with a silken rope, at Tyburn. She went to the execution of course, it could hardly be missed by those of the ton, and her friends and enemies noticed that she was 'Acting over all the old comedy of eyes' with a sometime lover. By now there must have been little left of her but those famous eyes. White lead poisoning had done for her, and she travelled to her home at Croome Court, near Worcester. Celebrated beauties die hard. Through the summer she lay on her sofa, watching the transformation of the parkland, which Coventry was laying out in the approved manner of the time. Her husband was absent, dabbling in politics in London. Her perpetual attitudes, her crowd of lovers, and her immense vanity had probably vanquished his affection. Besides, he had married the belle of her times, and such creatures are not expected to grow old, or ill, or to die.

She was attended by Doctor Wall of Worcester, whose spare time and money were taken up with the manufacture of porcelain, and whose exquisitely painted designs must have been an ironic reflection of those weeks with Lady Coventry, for paint was her only remaining interest. She would, we are told, lie for hours, looking into her mirror and recognizing real or imagined blemishes. As her face withered in the final few days of her life, she ordered her room to be darkened, and in that time, nobody saw her face.

She died on October 1st, and ten thousand people went to her country funeral. It was accepted that she died 'a victim to Cosmetics', and as a final touch of satire, the other character in the eighteenth century of whom this was said was Kitty Fisher, the actress-courtesan, who went the same way, killed by lead poisoning in 1767.

Ruined skins were one terrifying result of applied white lead paint; another was baldness, for hair fell out in handfuls after over-application, and for a time it became fashionable to shave the front of the hairline, probably because so few ladies had hair there anyway.

In pursuit of this fashion, children's foreheads were covered with walnut oil to decrease the growth of hair, and eyebrows were shaved ruthlessly. There were other methods of depilation. Plasters were the most common and painful remedy, and other hair removers were based on quick lime.

Horace Walpole gossips about the Duchess of Newcastle, who had a well-known beard. Her husband supposedly spent four hundred pounds with a French barber in his attempts to erase her hair, and when he left politics Walpole says: 'The Duke of Newcastle is retired . . . and will let his beard grow as long as his Duchess's.'

Although eyebrows were shaved they were replaced. The false eyebrow could be any colour and it could be placed anywhere, which accounts for the permanently surprised expression in some family portraits. The falsies were of mouse-skin, and the real eyebrow, after shaving, was obliterated with pink paste. Swift mentions:

> Her eyebrows from a mouse's hide
> Stuck on with art on either side.

And in *The Tender Husband* Steele declaims: 'Prithee Wench, bring me my black eyebrows out of the next room . . . no hang it, I'll wear these I have on.' This was in 1705, but the fashion was to persist until the extinction of artificiality at the end of the 1780s.

The natural eyebrow was blackened with a lead comb. During the century other methods would appear, they could be 'blackened with Gall water then brushed with a solution of green vitriol and gum arabic'. This 'doll' look may have come from Germany. At the court of Hanover women had the monotony of Mrs Noah, according to Lady Mary Wortley Montague who visited it in 1716, and judged those hefty mistresses who would have so much power when George I introduced them to England.

All the women have literally rosy cheeks, snowy foreheads and bosoms, jet eyebrows and scarlet lips to which they generally add coal black hair. These perfections never leave them until the hour of their deaths, and have a very fine effect by candlelight; but I could wish they were handsome with a little more variety. They resemble one another as much as Mrs. Salmon's Court [the contemporary waxworks], and are in as much danger of melting away from too near approaching the fire, which they do for that reason carefully avoid, though it is now such excessive cold weather that I believe they suffer greatly by that piece of self denial.

George I's favourite was the redoubtable Kielmansegge, later Countess of Darlington, who was described by Walpole: 'Large fierce eyes rolling beneath lofty arched eyebrows, two acres of cheeks spread with crimson, an ocean of neck that overflowed and was not distinguishable from the lower part of the body, and no portion of which was restrained by stays'.

He was later to describe Lady Mary Wortley Montague in terms as cruel as those she employed on the Germans, for after the ravages of smallpox she took to ceruse and Spanish wool with as much alacrity as anybody else; and by 1740 when the once sprightly girl had reached fifty-one: 'Her face is swelled violently on one side, with the remains of a [gummata], partly covered with a plaister, and partly with white paint, which for cheapness she has brought so coarse, that you would not use it to wash a chimney.'

The gummata to which Walpole so decorously refers may have been caused by syphilis or smallpox, but it was more probably brought about by the universally used mercurial wash, which was supposed to improve the complexion but generally eroded it. The best complexion milks were still those that were made out of simple herbal and floral mixtures, with no chemical contents. The aspiring country girls had more opportunities than the smart misses of St James's to collect cowslips, bladderwort, hartshorn or elder.

These treatments also sound alarming when one reads of the other ailments which might be healed by a flower, and considers that a purgative or scourer might not be the best base for a skin lotion. *The English Physician* was in every literate home. It would be thumbed over by the daughters of the family, the simple indexing of 'beauty lost' leads you to the ingredients. Thistles amend the rank smell of the armpits, and indeed the whole body and your urine. The seed of the common wild rocket 'mixed with honey, and used on the face, cleanseth the skin from morphew, and other Discolourings therein; and used with Vinegar, taketh away Freckles and Redness in the Face, or other Parts; and with the Gall of an Ox it mendeth foul scars, black and blue Spots, and the Marks of the Small-pox.'

These receipts, arising from the century-old *Gerard's Herbal* and the family doctrines of previous centuries, were to hold good until mass-advertising and the growth of brand names persuaded young girls that they would find a more swift and lasting beauty through goods bought in a shop.

It was part of the new conception of leisured society that there was now a special room in which to dress and make up. The advent of powder accelerated this notion. By the 1740s it became essential for an exquisite of either sex to have a powder closet or dressing room. The most elegant homes had them earlier than this date, as we can see in *The Rape of the Lock* or in Swift's cruel poem *The Lady's Dressing Room* written in 1730, and containing home truths about the usual state of the offices:

> Now listen while he next produces
> The various combs for various uses,
> Fill'd up with dirt so closely fixt
> No brush could force a way betwixt;
> A paste of composition rare,
> Sweat, dandruff, powder, lead and hair . . .
> There nightgloves made of Tripsey's hide,
> Bequeathed by Tripsey when she di'd;
> Here galley pots and vials plac'd,
> Some fill'd with water, some with paste;
> Some with pomatums, paints and slops,
> And ointments good for scabby chops.
> Hard by a filthy basin stands,
> Foul'd with the scouring of her hands;
> The basin takes whatever comes,
> The scrapings of her teeth and gums:
> A nasty compound of all hues,
> For here she spits and here she spues.

Celia, the unfortunate girl whose lover explored her dressing room in her

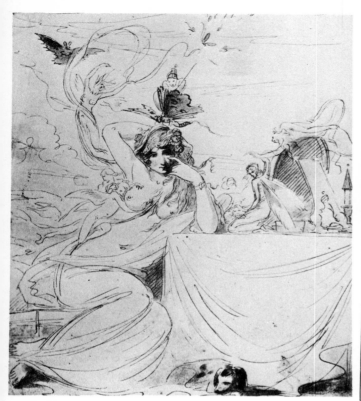

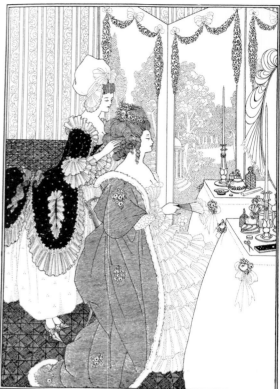

absence, also had a magnifying mirror in which she see the tiniest worm to be squeezed from her face; the final indignity for a beauty is her 'cabinet to vulgar eyes', the concealed chamber pot. Her lover is embarrassed and angry for he had hardly imagined:

> Such order from confusion sprung,
> And gaudy tulips rais'd from dung.

Steele, another exact chronicler, published in the *Tatler* a spoof advertisement for recovery of a dressing chest. 'Also a small cabinet, with six drawers inlaid with red tortoiseshell, and brass gilt ornaments at the four corners, in which were two leather forehead cloths, three pair of oiled dogskin gloves, seven cakes of superfine Spanish wool, half a dozen of Portugal dishes, and a quire of paper from thence; two pair of brand new plumpers, four black lead combs, three pair of fashionable eyebrows, two sets of ivory teeth, little worse for wearing, and one pair of box [wood] for common use . . . a spong dipped in Hungary water, left but the night before by a young lady going upon a frolic incog . . . together with receipts to make paste for the hands, pomatums, lip salves, white pots, beautifying creams, water of talk, and frog spawn water . . . and an approved medicine to procure abortion.'

This compendium was a travelling case of everything a beauty needed for her journeys to the waters, the country or the town. Forehead cloths were simply leather bands, impregnated with oil or grease which were bound round the head at night to smooth away lines. Dogskin gloves, like those made of poor Tripsey, were considered superior to ordinary leather ones, and they were also lined with oil and worn at night to smooth the hands. Spanish wool was the widely used red 'what the French call rouge', and it was not confined to

Far left Benjamin West *Belinda's Toilet c.* 1770 Pope's *Rape of the Lock* was illustrated by many later artists. Here, as visualized by a painter popular at the end of the eighteenth century.

Left Aubrey Beardsley *Belinda's Toilet* 1896 Beardsley imagined Belinda's dressing table as a fantasy of the taste of his own day, with flounces and ornaments reminiscent of those of a courtesan of the Belle Epoque.

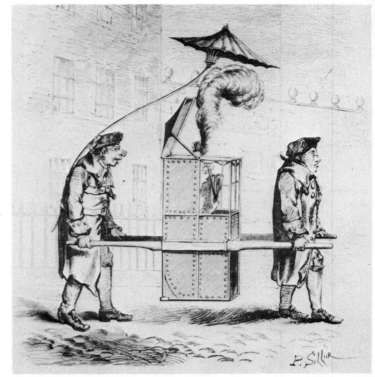

Right: A Fashionable Beauty on her Way to the Ball engraving by Sellier after James Gillray. 1796

ladies, as we have seen. Neither was it restricted to the cheeks. 'I hate this red stuff upon my lips', cries the playwright Mrs Centlivre in the *Platonick Lady* of 1706, 'I can't forbear licking 'em and it may be poison for aught I know.' There are even allusions to scarlet fingers, but no clue about the paintwork.

The plumper survived; it was a cork ball which swelled the cavities left by the loss of teeth. It had its stablemate in the Bosom Friend, a pad to make the breasts more full and nubile.

The breast was the vogue of the eighteenth century as surely as the rump enlarged by the bustle would become the zone of late Victorian attention, and the leg would symbolize the 1940s. Palpitating, hardly concealed, and covered with white powder from the age of fourteen, the skin of the most fashionable bosom was scabrous with inflammation, caused not only by the ceruse and chalk with which it was covered, but also by the continual descent of more powder and greasy pomatum from the hair.

In 1752 it was thought that 'the fashion is now to shew as low as one possibly can', but as the century passed, necklines slipped lower, although they were covered with muslin fichus out of some pretence of modesty. Walpole saw his first bosom bottle in 1754; 'a tin funnel covered with green ribbon' which held water for a posy.

Hairstyles and breasts made faces diminish in importance.

> One, two, nay, three cushions, like Cybele's towers;
> Then a few ells of gauze, and some baskets of flowers

said a contemporary poet of a barber's creation, hardly foreseeing that in the next decade the immense barrage balloon of hair would triumph over the body.

By 1760 the frivolity of make-up was established. Cosmetics had become a big business and the extravagance between the middle of the century and the *volte-face* of the French Revolution was to become so exaggerated that in comparison the early years of the century seemed almost innocent.

79

10 The Frenchwoman; and the Italianate man

At Versailles . . . the princesses wore it very brightly and very high in colour; they required that the rouge of women presented at court be more accentuated than usual on the day of their presentation . . . It was so widely demanded that in June 1780 a company offered five millions in cash to obtain the privilege of selling a rouge superior in quality to all kinds of rouge hitherto known. And in the following year Chevalier d'Elbée, who evaluated the annual sale at more than two million pots, asked that a tax of twenty five sols be imposed on each pot, to form pensions in favour of the wives and widows of impoverished officers.

So say the brothers Goncourt, writing in *The Woman of the Eighteenth Century*.

The French face of the period outdid all the others. Not only because more time and trouble was taken in France than elsewhere, but because cosmetics became a passion for their own sake, another piece of artistic artifice over which beauticians could pore for as much time as the jewellers would spend on the creation of boxes to hold the paint and powder. The French painters who catalogued this society had the most casual artifice of all. The trembling silvery skins in their portraits had the faintest hue of blue to suggest the presence of cosmetics and, unlike the English painters, they reproduced all the skill used by their sitters. (See page 104.)

Perhaps the truth was that the French were not ashamed of cosmetics and the English were. Multitudinous prints and paintings show French women in postures that were impossible in polite English portraiture . . . in bed, before the dressing table, even sitting on a bidet. They did not satirize cosmetics and other artifices, they applauded them. The shepherdesses who hardly sullied their white satin shoes in real grass, would wear rouge and ceruse without ever considering it an anachronism, but not the Englishwoman. If she is seen frowsty, dishevelled or cosmeticized it is in a caricature. Polite fiction maintained that the English gentlewoman had a superb natural complexion with no trace of the smallpox scars, and no record of the patches and paint that we know she really wore.

English portrait painters had established a convention. Sitters were not made up . . . this would appear to be the flattering invention of a bad portrait painter who might logically endow his patroness with a childlike complexion, but in fact the reverse is true. In bad paintings women are as doll-like as they must have appeared in reality, with red cheeks, black brows and porcelain skins . . . in fact, Lady Mary's German puppets. The great painters of the calibre of Reynolds and Gainsborough produced improbable sylphs, with blushes which appear more grateful to dew-dabbling than Spanish wool. By the same token, Gainsborough took liberties in showing the dresses of his sitters, and so women who were extravagantly jewelled and tightly corsetted appear in diaphanous gowns which are suggested rather than deciphered. It was a waste of money to pay a dressmaker if you wanted a good portrait.

Even Gainsborough was rebuked in 1772 for departing from the convention and for using 'too glowing colours' in comparison with Reynolds who used more subtle shades. In 1778 he produced three portraits for the Royal Academy of women of the demi-monde and drew this comment from the *Morning Chronicle*:

They are very fit subjects for Mr. Gainsborough's pencil, since he is rather apt to put that sort of complexion upon the countenances of his female portraits which are laughingly called in the School for Scandal as 'coming in the morning and going away at night' than to blend properly speaking, Nature's own red and white.

The face of the period was becoming more informal than it had been in the early years of the century. Goddesses were less fashionable than they had been when the Misses Gunning took society by storm. By 1783 the Duchess of Devonshire is the mode, with a snub nose, flyaway hair and wide grey eyes, characterized by 'hoydenish affability'. (See page 101.) Her charm relied on personality not regularity of features, and as a coquette with a pedigree she

Left Thomas Gainsborough *Mrs Robinson as Perdita* 1781. Detail. Wallace Collection, London
'Perdita' Robinson depicted in the English style as a child of nature
Right L. Cournerie *Marie Antoinette* (1755-93) Detail. Wallace Collection, London

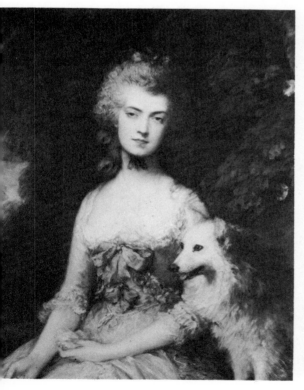

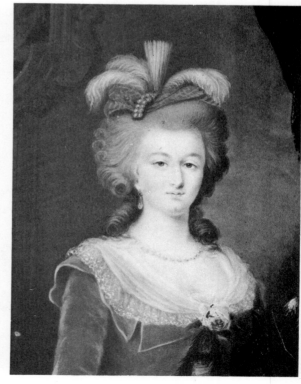

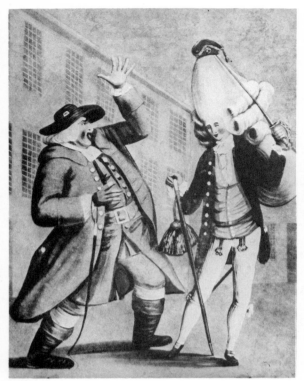
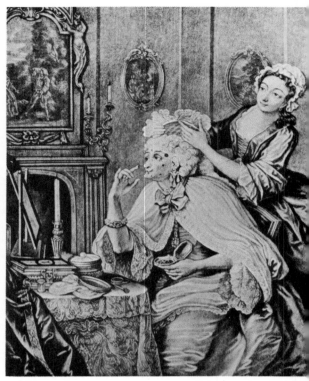

Left Grimm *'Well-a-day! Is this my son Tom?'* c. 1770
The advent of the Macaroni

Right: *Pride* engraving by James McArdell after C. A. Coypel, late eighteenth
century

succeeded where more clumsy Miss Hoydens would have failed. She is the
first intimation of the return to innocence, signalled before Rousseau and the
revolution. She also prefaced French fashions.

During the century France was establishing an ascendancy in fashion.
Louis XIV had pitifully striven to outdo his cousin Charles II without ever
appreciating that when Charles set the mode he was unaware of it. The
frenzy with which the French court attempted to outdo the English showed
results fifty years later. The court of the Hanovers could set new standards,
deficient though they might be in taste and innovation. The French had laid
the bedrock of a rigid school of fashion, and habits had been adopted which
could hardly be relinquished.

They were the acknowledged leaders of artificiality. The great royal
mistresses, Pompadour and Dubarry, had immense style, their scents of
patchouli and rose, and their ever-cascading ribbons, matched only by their
fountains, had set the scene for a beautiful queen. Marie Antoinette arrived
at court when she was fifteen and aroused immediate attention by her beauty.
Later, few writers could remember what was so particular about the young

girl, although some say her complexion, which is strange, for from her entrance on the French scene to her extraordinary exit, she wore heavy make-up. Baroness d'Oberkirch said of her: 'There are simply no words to give an idea of her dazzling complexion, literally a blend of lilies and roses. In her ash blonde hair swept up from a high forehead, there was only the faintest sprinkling of powder.' There were suggestions that the omission of powder was owing to a scalp or skin ailment.

The Americans were more discreet in their use of cosmetics. They continued to wear masks until the 'nineties. They also had their fashionable hairdressers but the mode was more restrained. The Americans seemed content to be provincial cousins who were bedazzled by the extremes of fashion in Europe when they visited it, but who were loath to make fools of themselves in front of their neighbours.

The advent of the Macaronis in the 'seventies was to be perpetually remembered by the Americans in *Yankee Doodle Dandy* but they were an emergent nation, involved in hazard during and after their war of independence, and therefore they had little time to ape the Europeans until they had become more established and wealthy, with an urban society.

The Macaronis themselves carried men's fashions and men's cosmetics to a new extreme.

They had been prefaced by the simple beaux of whom it was recorded in the *Connoisseur* of 1754 'they have their toilettes set out with washes, perfumes and cosmetics, and will spend a whole morning in scenting their linen, dressing their hair, and arching their eyebrows.' In spite of this spate of masculine arrogance, men remained fairly ingenuous in their use of fashion and cosmetics until the Macaronis arrived. They returned, in fact, from the Grand Tour which seems to have been the entrance ticket to the society, for initially they fostered Italian ideas and styles in London. Although the club was founded in 1764 it did not become the object of satire until the early 'seventies, when the mild and innocent passion for Italy had altered to an intense interest in exaggerated fashion, coupled with bad manners.

The *Town and Country Magazine* described them:

They make a most ridiculous figure with hats an inch in the brim, that do not cover but lie upon the head, with about two pounds of fictitious hair formed into what is called a 'club' hanging down their shoulders. The end of the skirt of their coat reaches the first button of their breeches which are either brown striped or white; their coat sleeves are so tight that they can with difficulty get their arms through their cuffs . . . their legs are covered with all the colours of the rainbow. Their shoes are scarce slippers and their buckles are within an inch of the toe. Such a figure, essenced and perfumed with a bunch of lace sticking under its chin, puzzles the common passenger to determine the thing's sex.

The writer must have seen enough painted men in his time to accept the rouge and powder of the Macaroni, what the commentators of the time found unendurable was this 'thing's' affectations. Every elegant man had a pad of Spanish wool upon his dressing table. In 1755 the *Connoisseur* had allowed that the masculine ruddy countenance was owing to its application. The Macaroni and his partner, the fop, were castigated for crimes of affectation, and not without cause. The worst of the Macaronis were credited with slitting watch-men's noses, and the best were capable of turning heads in the street.

> Soft silky coxcombs full of nice punctilio
> All paste, pomatum, essence and pulvilio
> With huge bouquets, like beaupots, daily go,
> Tricked out like dolls to pace the Rotten Row

wrote George Coleman in 1772.

Although they were derided as homosexual in intent, one of their main failings in the public eye was their success as seducers. Macaronis also worried their contemporaries by being inscrutable and languid. They are constantly depicted as being the cross an aged and respectable father had to bear. The continent received blame and condemnation for their behaviour, and they died away within a decade, leaving behind an attitude which remained as their signature. It is the Macaroni who heralds the quizzing glass and the high stock. His pretensions and exaggerations strayed into fashion and never really left it, for all his posturings with a cane or a glass, his attempts at wit (which in a Macaroni were merely rudeness) were to appear in the dandies from Brummell until the present day.

Many of their affectations seem pleasant to us. For instance, they adopted breath sweeteners and perfume, arousing normal gentlemen to declaim:

> I cannot talk with civet in the room
> A fine puss gentleman thats all perfume
> The sight's enough—no need to smell a beau
> Who thrusts his nose into a raree show?

In spite of this growl, men were becoming more aware of the pleasures of cleanliness. There were public baths in London and although soap and perfume were too expensive for the majority of people, a young buck would pride him-self on the ostentation of keeping clean. In 1765 he would go to the Hummums in Covent Garden, at the corner of Great Russell Street, where a gentleman might bathe, sup and sleep with a harlot for six guineas a night. Not one of your common harlots either, but a slap-up fashionable one, with little except her perfume to distinguish her from a real lady.

Courtesans were not only more sanitary than most ladies, they had discovered that business was better if they used breath sweeteners. At this period they were made of wine, bramble leaves, cinnamon, cloves, orange peel, burnt alum, gum lague and honey mixed with burnt ashes, and even if it ultimately pro-duced rot, it immediately produced a fine sweet breath. If you had patience to concoct the mixture, a tooth whitener could be made of lemon juice and burnt alum which was rubbed on to the teeth with a rag wound round a stick; and Chesterfield advised his son to clean his teeth often.

The continuing fashion for toothpicks, of coral, bone or simple wood, created a demand for toothpick cases, which were ornamented with jewels and carving. The fashionable young man, even if he were neither Macaroni or fop, had to carry a multiplicity of objects by the 1770s. They included patchboxes, snuff-boxes, toothpicks and two watches, one for show, and one to tell the time.

Ladies continued to wear false eyebrows, and a cosmetic shop displayed as a background to an advertisement of the 1780s proudly presents those of mouse-skin as a speciality. They were so obviously common knowledge that a lady at the theatre would adjust them with aid of a mirror concealed in her snuffbox, but a gentleman who cried out to his wife in an Assembly that her eyebrows were slipping, was rewarded by violent screams and she was carried into an outer room with a fit of hysterics.

Plumpers were still inserted into cavernous cheeks. 'Mrs. Button' says Mrs Cowley in *The Belles' Stratagem* '. . . wears cork plumpers in each cheek and never hazards more than six words for fear of shewing them.' This was in 1780.

Anticipating the revolution in politics, the revolution in English dress arrived, and with it the changing attitude to make-up. It is almost impossible to define the beginnings of the new ideal, though it owed a good deal to the Duchess of Devonshire's softened hair and piquante style and as much to the mature Marie Antoinette. The first bastion to fall was white hairpowder. The sprinkling of gold which was used by the French queen became currency in England. 'What do you think is the reigning mode in colour?' wrote Hannah More. 'Only turmeric, that coarse dye which stains yellow. It falls out of the hair and stains the skin so that every pretty lady must look yellow as a crocus.' White paint was disappearing, 'a little rouge is very pardonable but white paint is now looked on as disgraceful and dangerous', dictated the *Ladies' Magazine* in 1784.

In the *New Bath Guide* of 1776 Christoper Anstey, who was an acute social observer even if he was not a good poet, lists the necessities for a dressing table, and ceruse does not appear, although perfumes have become all important:

> Bring, o bring thy essence pot,
> Amber musk and bergamot,
> Eau de Chipre, eau de luce
> Sanspareil and citron juice
> Earrings, necklaces, aigrets,
> Fringes, blondes and mignionets,
> Fine vermillion for the cheek
> Velvet patches à la Grecque . . .

This is a foretaste. The rage for classical design hadn't arrived, but already patches had been worn with feeling. Fashion was to become an extension of emotion. The negligée had overcome the panniered dress. When stays were discarded it was sometimes unfortunate, for 'undress' was the great new look. It was some time before it was accepted. The blousiness of the new chemise style made it attractive in young ladies but fatal in their mothers. Many Englishwomen felt naked without the pannier and skins scored by years of addiction to ceruse could hardly be exposed to daylight. Yet miraculously, the right face and figure always appears when a fashion is accepted and just as square shoulders suddenly materialized in the 1940s, so lissom bodies appeared in the 1780s. It was hard to wear white, which was now the only possible colour, brought over from the West Indies in a wave of enthusiasm for the fine muslins. When pallor became the fashion ruddy French ladies had applied leeches to reduce their blood and then fainted away becomingly in company. The only thing which was not white was the head. The fichu, the straw hat, the flat shoes were all frames for a complexion of childhood. The 3000 hairstyles of Paris were reduced to one, with girlish curls framing the face.

The blonde became a beauty, and red hair, which had been considered unfortunate for the whole century, was now thought to be charming.

As if presaging the blow of the revolution, English, as well as French, society attempted to appear simple and rural. For a year before the revolution dress became childlike, and little girls and their mothers wore identical gowns. Their skins were clear, their eyes untouched by paint. Naturalism had set in.

But this return to nature had its own attendant problems. Skin tonics of every sort became important and the chemical lotions which replaced patch boxes and false eyebrows on the dressing table were as expensive as more blatant cosmetics.

At the beginning of the century the panacea had been Chymical Wash Balls, and the other purge-all of the century was the Barbaric Coroborant. It was also called a syrup for the preservation of long life. The Barbaric Coroborant had antecedents as grand as any duke's. The prevailing legend was that it had been discovered in Barbary by an Englishman serving there in the army of Charles V. As this king died in 1558 it gave some chronology to the lotion, which served the Englishman well until he was ninety-two, and then he willed it to the prebend of Canterbury. He in turn gave the recipe to the Countess of Feversham, and as The Countess of Feversham's Lotion it was widely sold during the eighteenth century. The recipe was published in every advice book of the period. It had to be made in May, and it included white wine, borage juice, flower de lis and gentian roots, all pounded together and reduced by simmering for twenty-four hours. This aristocratic compound was a great deal more innocent than that composed at this time by the mother of the Countess of Thanet, who fed a man with curious herbs intent on killing him, distilling him, and feeding the potion to her husband.

Freckles were still anathema, and ointments to reduce them included a wash of wood ash, strawberries, grapejuice and asses' milk. One ointment included lead sulphate which probably removed the skin immediately.

All these potions for fresh complexions also offered far more. By the age of naturalism, fashionables were demanding more than a promise of good skin, they wanted to know about chemical properties, about electricity in the body and the chances of potency and longevity.

The ointment merchants pandered to them mercilessly. A first-class potion would make you live forever and also turn you into a beauty. The advertisement for Chymical Wash Balls is harmless compared with the claims made by cosmeticians, who were also almost magicians, such as Cagliostro.

This intelligent Italian arrived in London in 1776 with his wife, Seraphina. He was a great public relations expert, and his advertisement was always for himself. The self-appointed count travelled with a black japanned box painted over with cabalistic signs and Masonic symbols. He wore a blue fox greatcoat and perfumed the air about him. Cagliostro was not mean in recounting his experiences, for he had seen the building of the ark and the crucifixion, and he had been an initiate of the temple of Solomon. He preached Rosicrucianism, of which he was the Grand Master. He is still a mystery. It is certain that he had tremendous magnetism and that his teachings were potent enough to influence Goethe and Schiller. Dumas felt that he was the prime architect of the French Revolution, but in 1776 Cagliostro was grubbing for a living in Whitcombe Street, Soho. His wife was amazingly beautiful and she remained his chief publicity. Seraphina was also Italian, her real name was Lorenza, but for her husband's purposes she had no nationality. He seems to have persuaded his public that Seraphina was of another world than this, and her blonde, cool beauty aroused the interest of London society:

Duels were fought on the subject of the colour of Countess Cagliostro's eyes or whether the dimple was in her left cheek or her right. When she rode out on her black stallion, Djerid, her ardent admirers rushed to see her pass.

When he set up shop in France, 500 customers a day came to Cagliostro. He would lay on his hands and cure the sick; but ten years before, in London, he had not gained that stature. His Soho shop was a mixture of chemist and necromancer, presided over by the mysterious Seraphina. The count, who was small and thick-set with an olive skin, could woo the the most disaffected stranger with a voice like that of trumpet, harsh, metallic and persuasive.

The best-selling article in his London shop was Beautifying Water, although Wine of Egypt sold well, intended to aid the man whose natural appetites were slipping away. Cagliostro knew the virtue of expense and sold his Egyptian Pills for thirty shillings a dram. But his beauty shop was not a success and his career as a magician had hardly begun, before he was deported abruptly by the police for selling fake lottery tickets. He returned when he was deported from France in 1786, for his role in the affair of the queen's necklace, and rented an apartment at 4 Sloane Street. He was a compulsive wanderer and perhaps he found that the air in London was not sympathetic to a man who had been so closely involved with the most celebrated crime of the period.

The post-revolution simplicity emphasized basic physical problems, for instance, the green pallid skins of the girls during the Napoleonic wars suggest that their diets were deficient, but at least their skins were not covered with killing cosmetics. Outside London habits died hard, and the prevalence of rouge continued; no elegant women would wear false colour during the Regency period, but it still seemed strange to older women to go about with naked faces. Ceruse was given its dismissal by a provincial paper in 1787 when the *Ipswich Journal* suggested that ladies who frequented Bath (and what real lady did not?) must beware: 'Those who use white paint as a cosmetic are liable to have their skins turn entirely yellow, if not black, from the phlogistic vapours which arise from the mineral springs.'

There was a momentary revival of rouge, 'natural complexions have been gradually on the decline among the ladies since the introduction of rouge and white lead', said the *Morning Post* of 1799 as if it were announcing a new innovation. The balance righted itself, for presently ladies used a little colour if they chose and fashion altered with every season, although that fine hectic flush would never entirely reappear.

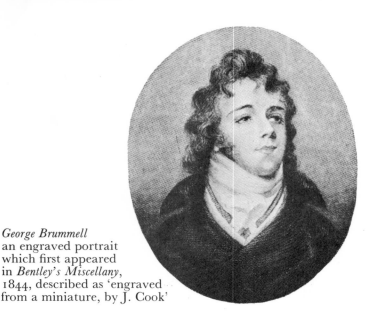

George Brummell
an engraved portrait
which first appeared
in *Bentley's Miscellany*,
1844, described as 'engraved
from a miniature, by J. Cook'

11 The Regency dandy

While women exiled themselves from fashion by adhering to the simplicity of innocence, men achieved more distinction in their dress and manners. It was a masculine age in Britain between 1790 and 1840. The women who became notable were those sharp-eyed and -tongued novelists such as Fanny Burney, and later, Jane Austen and Maria Edgeworth; or the demi-mondaines like Harriet Wilson whose memoirs convulsed a nation.

The leader of the revolution, which was as dramatic in dress as it was in politics, was George Bryan Brummell. As we have seen, the taste for white had already been admitted but it had hardly spread among men with the same alacrity as it had with women. The stories of this young man's influence were exaggerated, but denoted the surprise with which cleanliness and a sober taste in dress were received in England. His audacity was amazing, and endeared him to the Prince Regent exactly as it would alienate him from him in later years. Instead of playing down his humble ancestry Brummell vaunted it; yet owing to his father's success as a civil servant he went to Eton, where he had an early reputation as an eccentric and wit. He left Oxford after a few months, on inheriting a vast fortune, suggested at between fifteen to sixty-five thousand pounds; and he enrolled in the army, becoming an officer in a crack regiment with the usual passport of the period—a bought commission and an understanding that he could support himself as a officer in a way which would redound to the regiment's vanity. Two years later Brummell was the intimate friend of the future George IV, translated there by some alchemy of temperament. To the indignation of the prince's wife, Caroline, Brummell had an ascendancy which precluded anybody else's influencing George. He was the most fashionable figure of the day, spending his time between White's and Brookes' and interminable house parties. He became the arbiter of ton society, or the fashionable world. Duchesses could be brought down by a slighting word from him, and an obscure young man would achieve instant success after walking with Brummell in the park. He ruined himself by taking the part of

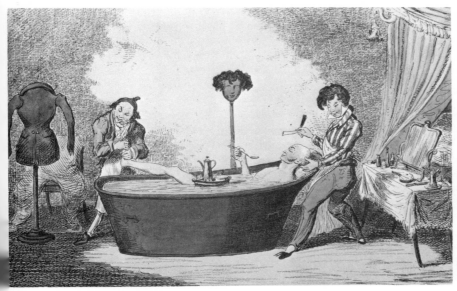

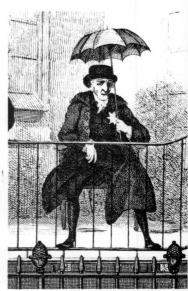

Left Diogenes Tiger *Parisian Luxury* 1824
The age of the ascetic beau had passed and the dandies of the post-Napoleonic
period were resplendent with colour and scents.

Right : Old Q on the Balcony
Celebrated as a rake, Old Q collected girls from his balcony viewpoint.

Maria Fitzherbert in her altercations with the Prince Regent, and when that
stout party became king, Brummell, like Falstaff, was dismissed; and he
consoled himself by gambling his money away. He disappeared overnight in
1816, to live a dull existence in France until 1840, finally losing his job as consul
at Caen, and ending as a senile, uncouth and shabby old man. But Brummell
in his early years lit a lamp for fashion which was never dimmed. His immacu-
late linen and superlative clothes made him the object of satire, but also of
admiration, His valet's descent from the bedroom with an armful of cravats
was explained simply: 'These,' he said, 'are our failures.'

Until Brummell's day many men had assumed that deshabille suggested
aristocratic ways, and the previous arbiters of fashion—relieving themselves
at public chamber pots, wearing spurs in the drawing room and spitting on the
floor—were discountenanced by Brummell's behaviour. He even cleaned his
teeth, saying to his audience of young bucks: 'Oh there's a spot—ah! it's
nothing but a little coffee. Well, this is excellent powder, but I won't let any of
you have the receipt for it.' His shaving was sublime, and his clean face abashed
the bluebeards about St James's. His ablutions went on for hours, with alternate
immersions and scrubbings. He would finally scrub his face with a rough
brush, until the circulation was pounding, and then would stand with a mirror
picking out any hairs left on his face with a pair of tweezers. He always wore
plain fabrics, with a blue coat and buff breeches. The soles of his sleek-fitting
boots were polished to a uniform black with the uppers; and his linen, lightly
starched and carefully wound, was always spotless. The true character of
Brummell was succeeded by many distorted fictional portrayals of the dandy,
one of the most famous of which was Pelham in Bulwer Lytton's novel of the
same name, published in 1828. Pelham was not as suave as a real dandy. His
mannerisms were absurd, and perpetuated a myth of languor which was not
necessarily true of the living dandies, who spared no effort in achieving their
own perfection. Pelham had perfumed curtains, and used eau-de-cologne.

Anticipating the young man of Huysman's *A Rebours,* he wished to have each course in a meal served with a different perfume.

In the 1820s the cool dandy was ousted by D'Orsay, a perfumed, ruffled, pastel-hued creation with punctiliously waved auburn sidewhiskers. The painter Benjamin Robert Haydon described him as having a white greatcoat, blue satin cravat, hair oiled and curling, hat of the primest curve and purest water, gloves scented with eau-de-cologne, or eau-de-jasmine, primrose in tint, skin in tightness . . . 'His beauty is that of a rather disgusting sort which seems to be . . . of no sex,' wrote Jane Welch Carlyle. If she found him repulsive, many did not and were enraptured by his addiction to the dressing table.

A new voluptuary had taken the place of the old rogues of the Regency and the usurper was to be superseded in Britain by the black broadcloth and scrubbed face of the Victorian divine, whether he was a squire, a businessman, or a politician. The young Disraeli held out against the abiding passion for sobriety, but even he succumbed, although he did not cut off his ringlets or eliminate dye from his hair. No tales would be told of the Victorian sybarites like those which circulated about the wicked Duke of Queensberry, who sat in his window overlooking Green Park eyeing every pretty passer-by. He bathed in milk, said the whispered legends, and one eye was of glass.

The dandies bought their paints in Bond Street, the men's shopping area until the end of the nineteenth century. Ladies 'went to stores in Oxford Street where there were five perfumers listed in *Johnson's Commercial Guide* for 1817; the city was gaslit in the early years of the century and some attempts were being made by shops to woo out-of-town customers who could hardly ask for lip salve or rouge in their own country market towns but who might approach a sympathetic shop assistant in the city with equanimity, or even send for goods from a country address. The shop assistant has been an unknown factor in the sale of cosmetics, yet the wise early-nineteenth-century proprietors knew the value of the handsome young man with glossy black whiskers and an elegant waistcoat, who could gain the confidence of ladies and ever-so-discreetly flirt with them. In 1806 the *Morning Chronicle* was to inveigh against them:

> A soft automatum in shape of man
> Powder'd and perfumed, see the creature stalk,
> Smile like a lady, delicately talk,
> Choose out a headdress, praise lace shifts to sin in,
> Or descant on the prettiest baby linen;
> Commend the muslin drawers, or advise
> The pillowy shape to swell the female size.

Three years before, the same journal had issued an invective against the beaux of Bond Street who blanched their hands with whiteners and made their cheeks brown with walnut juice. This was an unusual fashion, for other observers noticed the prevalence of rouge among those gentlemen who had not yet been influenced by Brummell. In 1808, the satirist commented that the dandy wore a perpetual blush. The problem of the age was over-indulgence and in the matter of rouge the men went at it as they went at jumps on their steeplechasers, from the 1780s until the realization that it was outmoded.

Some of them did not realize that they were out of date until the year of Waterloo, although the Prince Regent himself, affected by his close friendship with the exquisite mentor, used leeches to decrease his florid complexion. His habits were gravely altered by Brummell, for in 1822 his perfumery bill went down to £263 a year, but when the favourite was outcast, it amazingly rose again, to £500 17s. 11d. in 1828.

Most of this perfume was eau-de-cologne, under the benign influence of Brummell. George's natural appetite was for flowery smells but the beau dictated that perfume was unnatural on a man, and that his linen should merely smell of the open air, as it should be sent to Hampstead for laundering, where it could dry on the Heath. In spite of his doctrines, men continued to use Hungary water, rosewater, imperial water (made of mastic, pine nuts, frank-incense, cloves and benzoin, and suitable as a mouth wash), and honey waters, which included orange-flower water, vanilla and musk.

Eau-de-cologne was a fairly new fashion. It had originally been called Aqua Mirabilis and had been the inspired product of the Farina brothers, who were Italian silk dealers in Cologne. They had introduced the perfumed water as a sideline in their shop. When Cologne was inundated by foreign troops in the Seven Years War, they did a roaring trade and their toilet water spread over Europe. In England it even served as a pick-me-up after a drunken night, and Sheridan would tipple at eau-de-cologne judiciously mixed with brandy and arbusquade, which was a lotion put on shot wounds.

The ubiquitous cologne was to remain in many dressing rooms after all the other paints had disappeared; only the few sad relics of painted men continued until the young queen herself grew old. In 1877, Disraeli noted that Lord Malmesbury was skilfully rouged: 'People say that resource is effeminate. M. is manly enough, and the two most manly persons I ever knew, Palmerston and Lyndhurst, both rouged. So one must not trust too much to general observation.'

The aubade to cosmeticized men came with the passing of the Regency and those who persisted beyond that time were deliberately eccentric.

Generally the painted man had become despicable:

. . . a being in regard to appearance of very doubtful gender, laced up like a young lord, a pair of cossacks resembling a petticoat, a crop like a pouting pigeon, a painted face looking over a wall of starch and muslin, a patch at the corner of the mouth . . . the made-up male doll who when wig, dyed whiskers, stiff cravat, padded breast, corset, paint and perfume are taken away, sinks into something worse than nothing. (Captain McDonagh *The Hermit in London*,1822)

The made-up male doll was to be finally eclipsed by the fashions which came back from France. Brummell had his day in which the lean sleek line achieved a pre-eminence which was never really usurped in many masculine styles, but it had received a fillip from the fashions which emerged from Paris, when the triumphant British flocked there after the Napoleonic wars, to review the French styles from which they had been removed for so long. The Merveilleuses and Incroyables had made pallor fashionable and had only enhanced their natural appearance with sweet waters.

Languor was the true height of fashion and some determined characters even drank vinegar to achieve the reed-slim line of the die-away mode. During the aftermath of the revolution designs had been as indeterminate as one might expect in a country where nothing was stable or expected. A gibe at the most elegant stylists was made by the *Journal de Paris* on the 23 Mersidor, Year 11 when they introduced the term 'Sexa' for the most extravagant leaders of fashion, which was a supposed abbreviation of 'Qu'est-ce que c'est que ça?' The most exquisite men had a new device for beauty which even the most outrageous rouged dandies of London had never imagined. This was to have the optic nerve loosened, so that a quizzing glass became essential.

The quizzing glass certainly reached England after 1815, with devastating results, for it intimidated shopmen and servants, hypnotized the ladies, and gave the most refined gentlemen an excuse to know each other or not, as they wished. Everything was quizzed, from a pretty pair of ankles to one's dinner. It enraged the older men, for the support of a glass entailed an extortionate air of hauteur, which was quite insupportable. The dandy with the closely stayed figure, the full bosom, created by a small cushion, the carefully rumpled hair, enamelled face, and violet coat, made Regency London gay, if not pleasant. It was the last version of the painted man and it was a splendid, inconsequential one. The dandy would be superseded by the swell, and the swell by the masher, the chappie, the Piccadilly Johnnie, and the aesthete during the nineteenth century, but men would never have quite the same ridiculous panache.

The painted dandy disappeared from the London streets, but he was preserved in the army, for by the Crimean war a few of the high-ranking officers were still rouging their cheeks and clambering into stays; in a perverted sense the continuation of the ancient cosmetic fashions labelled them as roaring boys, sharp on the parade ground, devils in bed with a pretty woman, and capable of being six-bottle-a-night guests when they stayed with their antique friends in country houses. These pomatumed generals had little link with the Victorian age, they were relics of the most extravagant Regency bucks who had not been influenced by Brummell but who had been leftovers of an earlier bucks' society, and they were proud of their eccentricities.

In retrospect, the women of the Regency seem pale figures whose styles hardly altered from the French revolution until the advent of the young queen. In fact, the fashion in cosmetics was erratic, with rouge ebbing and flowing from season to season. Although Jane Austen herself was said to rouge, her heroines hardly did so, and while one feels that the rattling Lydia or imperious Maria might have dabbed at their cheeks with a rabbit's foot, the demure sardonic central characters put no more on their cheeks than a handkerchief, when it was raised to an eye, hiding laughter rather than tears. Ladies were hardly so demure in real life, for the dresses of the period were more daring than they had ever been before or have been since.

Muslin gowns exposed nude bodies beneath, and white was to remain the most sympathetic colour for many years. Its candour eliminated the class differences in dress, and the girl from a rich family was only removed from a cottager by the daring of her gown. The diaphanous dresses made any court occasion a randy event and when one magistrate heard that young ladies still wore Bosom Friends to aid their natural shape, he cried 'Thank heavens they still wear something!'

Harmony of colour was most important and so simple contrasts to white were almost the only permissible shades. This vogue for matching colours was to continue until the worst excesses of Victorian dress in the 1860s, and until then most women wore muted tones which blended together fortuitously. The

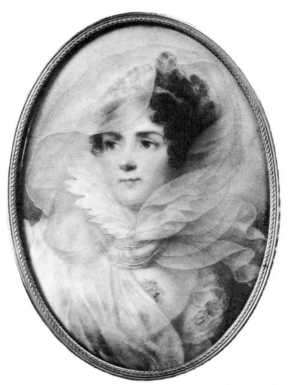

Jean Baptiste Isabey *The Empress Josephine* (1763-1814) Wallace Collection, London

thin dresses which were the vogue between 1800 and 1810 caused side effects of pneumonia and bronchitis, yet few girls discarded their simple classical gowns.

In France the new élite which succeeded the revolutionaries altered the romantic pallor. The prime instrument was Josephine herself, whose addiction to fashion had persisted throughout all the tribulations she had suffered before she married Napoleon. She was not pale and interesting but sallow, and perhaps influenced by memories of her old fashioned West Indian upbringing. She restored rouge and used it herself with prodigality . . . one year's supply cost the emperor more than three thousand francs.

The English girls too became quite ruddy. Caroline Burney's novel *Seraphina or a Winter in Town* was published in 1809, and she observed: 'They run about with hardly any clothes on, and their faces painted scarlet red.' In the same decade Susan Sibbold commented, 'To rouge was all the rage and without your cheeks were the colour of a peony you were not à la mode.' In 1806, *La Belle Assemblée* the critical ladies' magazine, said, 'On the toilet of our ladies the rouge box is become perhaps the most essential attendant.'

Maria Edgeworth saw the fashion in a different light. In *Belinda,* a novel published in 1801, she portrays the world through the eyes of a simple girl who is fascinated by high life when she stays with the devastating Lady Delacour for a London season. Belinda watches her hostess intently.

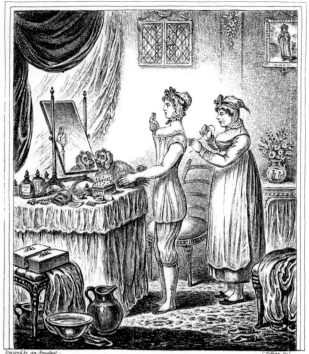

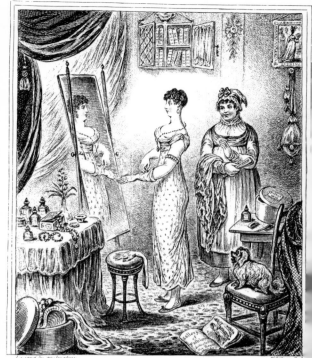

Progress of the Toilet. — THE STAYS. — Plate 1.
London Publish'd February 26th 1810 by H Humphrey 27 St James's Street

Progress of the Toilet. — DRESS·COMPLETED. Plate 3.
London Publish'd February 26th 1810 by H Humphrey. 27 St James's Street

James Gillray *The Progress of the Toilet* 1810

There had always been some mystery about her ladyship's toilette: at certain hours doors were bolted . . . Miss Portman at first imagined that Lady Delacour dreaded the discovery of her cosmetic secrets, but her ladyship's rouge was so glaring, and her pearl powder so obvious, that Belinda was convinced that there must be some other cause for this toilette secrecy.

When Lady Delacour visits Belinda and sees her bare dressing table: 'But you don't paint . . . no matter you will . . . you must . . . every body must, sooner or later,' she says cynically, having confided that she is in good spirits owing to a double dose of opium. Later she turns upon the girl, convinced that she is a rival, and produces a hysterical scene (after which she has to be rouged afresh):

'Miss Portman,' said her ladyship, turning carelessly towards her, 'where do you buy your rouge? . . . Lady Singleton, would you rather at this moment be mistress of the philosopher's stone, or have a patent for rouge that will come and go like Miss Portman's?—Apropos! Have you read St Leon?'

Lady Delacour is suffering from a wasting disease and so her ridicule and rouge are later considered equally appropriate.

Maria Edgeworth was a confirmed opponent of cosmetics, so much that she devoted a short story in her collection of *Moral Tales*, published in 1803, to a woman who suffered from their application.

Mrs. Ludgate caught a violent cold, and her face became inflamed and disfigured by red spots. Being to go to a ball in a few days, she was very impatient to get rid of the eruption; and in this exigency she applied herself to Mr. Pimlico the perfumer, who had often supplied her with cosmetics and who now recommended a beautifying lotion. This quickly cleared her complexion; but she soon felt the effects of her imprudence; she was taken dangerously ill, and the physician who was consulted attributed her disease entirely to the preparation she had applied to her face.

She recovers, but is filled with pique to discover that she is now no longer the belle of the neighbourhood.

Her vanity was deeply wounded; and her health appeared to her but a secondary consideration, in comparison with the chance of recovering her lost complexion. Mr. Pimlico who was an eloquent perfumer, persuaded her that her former illness had nothing to do with the beautifying lotion she had purchased at his shop; and to support his assertions, he quoted examples of innumerable ladies of high rank and fashion, who were in the constant habit of using this admirable preparation. The vain and foolish woman, notwithstanding the warnings which she had received from the physician who attended her during her illness listened to the oratory of the perfumer, and bought half a dozen bottles of another kind of beautifying lotion. The eruption vanished from her face, after she had used the cosmetic; and, as she did not feel any immediate bad effects upon her health, she persisted in the practice for some months. The consequence was at last dreadful. She was found one morning speechless in her bed, with one side of her face distorted and motionless. During the night she had been seized with a paralytic stroke: in a few days she recovered her speech; but her face continued totally disfigured.

It was not Maria Edgeworth's tales but the French fashion which resulted in the decline of rouge for women, as it had for men. They had other pleasures, such as chiropodists who came to the house and were able to perform their trade with a lady in a dressing gown, to the amusement of some husbands and the horror of others. They had wax bosoms made to swell their own when the dress styles altered to a more staid and contrived shape with slightly flared stiff skirts and pronounced bosoms and waists. A few ladies still wore cork plumpers but, like rouge, such obvious artifice was beginning to be *outré*. The forewarning of an innocent young queen altered the character of society. Innocence extended to modes of dress, for during the late 1820s women went to dinner parties in formal gowns with light veils over their bared shoulders, and they arrived with posies which stayed with them during the meal. A glass of water was placed on the table for each lady, so that 'the table looks like a bed of flowers'.

The general picture was important, for the shape was a new conception to the early Victorian women who adopted a neat, clean line in dress with exaggerated sleeves, modest necklines, arch little heads with descending corkscrew curls, and a skirt like an isosceles triangle, descending to neat little feet. Modesty had arrived, and cosmetics were to disappear, swept away by the enthusiasm for a natural mode which would be succeeded by a theory in which ugliness became a moral virtue.

12 The Victorian myth of womanhood

Perhaps the Victorian lady went to her chaise longue in defence against a moral decree which forbade any screen against the weather. She no longer wore a mask. Her face was naked and exposed. Only harlots and old-fashioned country women used lotions. It was a sign of virtue to have red roughened cheeks, and this exposure to cold, augmented by a diet which made the complexion spotted and sallow, may have resulted in the flurry with which the aristocracy and then the middle class took to their sofas, shielded from harsh light by velvet drapes or blinds. Few Victorians were seen closely in strong light once they had passed their youth. At night they were aureoled by oil lamps and gas lights; during the day they lay in semi-darkness. They undressed in the dark, the rich woman would breakfast in bed and come down to the main part of the house when her husband had left for his office, his club or his estate. Their lives were segregated against any intrusion of candour.

Their complaint was called the green sickness, because of the pallor which accompanied it. This term covered as many shades as the decline. It was no doubt the result of constipation, infrequent exercise and the mystery of femininity, for though their lives must have been ordered by pregnancy and menstruation, the Victorian lady never admitted her problems. When the townswoman of the 'sixties went shopping her face was shrouded by a bonnet and in later years she would have a veil. She was not alone. Behind her was a maid, or more usually a page boy or footman. In London she would leave him outside the shop and these uppity servants would congregate under the arcades of Regent Street while their mistresses made mysterious purchases from innocent stores. There were no beauticians, a perfumer might make up a perfume or the occasional lotion, but these preparations were bought with more alacrity by men, who would find them in their own shopping areas of Burlington Arcade and Bond Street. Hair dye was no doubt used by a few women, but it was advertised for men, along with pomatum, and Rowland's Macassar Oil, which passed forever into the language with the arrival of antimacassars.

The mode, celebrated by cartoonists as well as fashionable portrait painters, was the oval face, a pink and white complexion and a small rosy mouth. This tiny orifice, useless for anything except the emission of a sigh, had been popularized by the queen, who had been depicted by Winterhalter as a pouting cherub. Like Twiggy's flat breasts, the rosebud mouth might have been an infection spreading through the populace; Trollope's heroines had this minute mouth, and so did Little Nell. Eyes on the other hand were large, and often deep blue, set under elegant thin arched brows. In describing the Victorian face, novelists could expand, for they certainly could not describe any other part of anatomy unless it were 'the prettiest little foot in the world'.

The strict regime was reduced to absolute simplicity by Fanny Duberly writing to her sister from the Crimea and asking her to order from Savory and Moore some essentials which included:

96

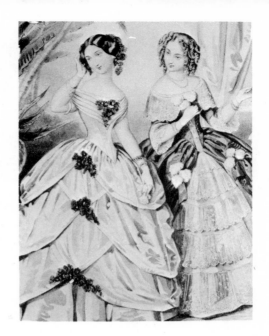

Le Follet fashion plate after Adèle Anais Toudouze *c.* 1853
The early Victorian ideal which can rarely have been attained in reality was the norm in fashion plates and illustrations to novels.

2 large bottles Marrow Oil
4 Bottles of Bandoline (Eau Lustrant)

The only aid to beauty which could be admitted was eau-de-cologne. Rimmels in the Strand sold perfumed gloves although these must have been for the demi-monde; their false violets had collapsible stems imbued with the smell of violets, one imagines these must have been tiny phials of scent which would create an aroma when the wearer was brushed in a waltz. How much more exciting if she were ever crushed in an embrace! The artificially enhanced violets could not have been intended for good women. Flaubert benefited from the use of eau-de-cologne. Having created the most feminine creature in literature, who had been entrapped by her own artifice, he objected to a girl he met on the train in 1869. She shared his carriage, smoked cigarettes and put her feet up on the seat; but as he felt faint, the cocotte offered him her eau-de-cologne and revived him.

The Victorian male remained in imagined or tactful ignorance about the smells of oris, patchouli and violets. He had his own scents. The heavy swell had taken the place of the true dandy, and he was a sporting man in voluminous trousers and draped with whiskers. The comic writers of the middle of the century saw the demise of artifice. The plaintive hero of Samuel Warren's *Ten Thousand a Year* tries to dye his hair with Cyanochaitanthropopiou, 'only seven and sixpence for the smaller sized bottle . . . one was in a twinkling placed upon the counter where it lay like a miniature mummy, swathed as it were, in manifold advertisements.' Alas, Titmouse's hair turns green and an application of Damascus cream turns it violet. He longs for it to be carroty once more and buys Tetrargmenon Abracadabra at Nine and Sixpence, which is perfectly colourless with an infernal smell; next morning his hair is purple and his whiskers are white. He has to enter high society in this peculiar fashion but he does attempt to remedy his problem with a pot of ostrich grease and rhinoceros marrow, 'the one being suet and the other lard, differently scented and coloured'.

Rouge was the viper. This one word described all the abhorred paint. When a comic writer introduces a character with rouge, they are damned as

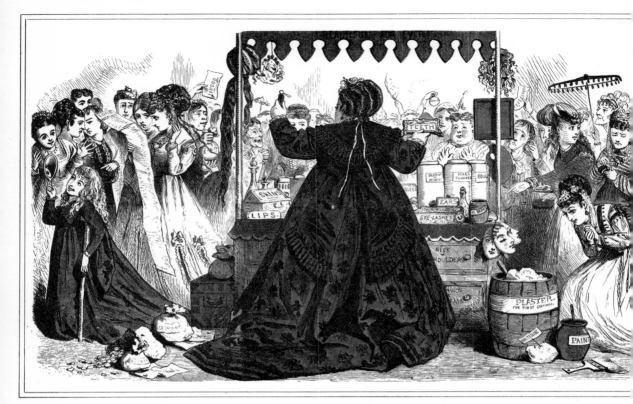

Vanity Fair c. 1870. In spite of the repeated assertions that 'nice girls' would not wear make-up, here is a parody of a cosmetician who delivers a remarkable range of goods.

immoral or eccentric. In *The Pottleton Legacy* Albert Smith created crazy old Lady Flokes. She was a pantomime dame of 1852, with 'a great quantity of cloudy lace and scarves of ancient splendour, rouged highly . . .' she also 'wore ringlets and carried a large flacon of salts'. When she introduced the gentle heroine to her room, there was 'by her patchbox, a book of Chinese rouge that looked green and rubbed crimson, which Lady Flokes was anxious to put aside'. Later in the same novel, Smith introduces another scandalous old lady, Mrs Must, and this anecdote:

she had been to town to have a tooth out, without pain, by the new discovery, and when the gentleman who operated put a damp cloth over her face to bring her round, he bought off all her rouge as well—a frightful thing—the old lady being of Lady Flokes's class and presumed never to wash, or if she did, to spend a more frightful sum on face plaster and red ochre generally than would have repaired and arabesqued her tumble-down conservatory.

The last relic of rouge was typically Victorian in concept for it was called 'the sympathetic blush' and so intended for those sigh-away evenings with the scent of crushed violets. This cream appeared white but contained alloxan, an oxide which turned pink when it had been exposed to the air. It created the same problems that instant suntan creams present today, in that the wearer could not estimate how rosy her face would appear a few hours later.

The Americans were now more adventurous. When Meg in *Little Women* is induced to try powder for a fashionable party it is not of course considered correct for a minister's daughter; but English girls in the same environment would not have had any access to cosmetics.

13 The end of Victorian morality

In America a spirit of levity had succeeded the Civil War. The pioneers could hardly worry about being circumspect, although in the east the same pallid complexions pertained as in England, there was a 'bounce' in fashion. The American upper classes visited Paris and noticed that artificial aids were used. When they visited the newly imported operas bouffes which Jay Fiske showed in his theatre, they daringly used a little powder and even lip rouge. It was as if an era of repression had ended, everything was turned topsy turvy, scandal was rife, with stories like Henry Ward Beecher's seduction of his friend's wife filling the pages of daily newspapers; and the elevation of unscrupulous *nouveaux riches* who liked their wives or mistresses to be 'well turned out' and who didn't mind dyed golden hair. The old aristocracy of America had little opportunity to inflict its European morals on the *arrivistes*. They were under siege themselves and had to conform to a cruder, ruder doctrine. The hostesses of New York had a racy bohemian attitude to ornament and Mrs Stuyvesant Fishe wouldn't turn a girl away from her vast soirées because she wore powder. The 'seventies were striving to assimilate so many new ideas and so many new territories that the painted ladies were acceptable. Harriet Hubbard Ayer instigated another breakthrough in the field of cosmetics.

Harriet Hubbard, an ungainly child, was married at the age of fifteen to Herbert Ayer, the eldest son of John Vanessa Ayer, an iron magnate. Harriet was allowed to be extravagant. Her father-in-law and her husband encouraged her to give magnificent dinner parties and to dress by Worth. Her visits to Paris resulted in an elegant way of life, and as she travelled and entertained, Harriet Ayer became a beauty with more intelligence than one might expect from a pretty dress-hanger.

Her marriage did not survive her way of life. Her husband spent less and less time at home, and as they became alienated, Harriet determined on divorce and left her fashionable home in Chicago. She took her children and rented an apartment in New York. Hardly had she done so, when Herbert, who was now head of the family, lost his money in speculation and so she was left a divorcee with a sense of style and no money. She supported her children by selling antiques for a furniture store and she became so successful that she was sent to Paris where furniture could be bought for the millionaire Americans. While she was there, Harriet had her face cream made up by a chemist and, on impulse she bought the prescription. She had already met Jim Seymour, a multi-millionaire broker who was prepared to back her in her own business.

It was 1886 and Harriet Hubbard Ayer estimated correctly that the climate was changing and that women would presently use face creams and even tinted cosmetics. Jim Seymour lent her 50,000 dollars. Her gambit was the first example of audacious advertising in this field. She based her campaign on the story that this was the cream used by Mme Récamier. This advertisement promised more than everlasting youth. It told a story, written by Harriet Hubbard Ayer herself:

How Julie Récamier preserved her beauty for over half a century
Julie Récamier was acknowledged for over forty years to be the most beautiful woman in France. Her loveliness was such a power that Napoleon once said of her, 'I fear Madame Récamier's influence more than the muskets of a whole army' . . . For over forty years the women of her most picturesque period marvelled and fruitlessly endeavoured to ascertain by what means Madame Récamier preserved her transcendently lovely complexion. The mystery was never revealed and it was by the merest accident I came into possession of the secret . . . While in Paris many years ago, I suffered from the effects of the sun and my complexion seemed irretrievably injured. I was stopping at a small private hotel and an old lady (the Countess de C.) sitting opposite me brought me a little pot containing a paste which she had used all her life, a compound made for the celebrated beauty, Julie Récamier.

The healing medical powers of the cream were underlined, as it was a spot remover. Even in the enlightened USA cosmetics could not be advertised as a means of attracting men. But it was probably the combination of 'story' advertisements and well-known figures that ensured the success of the Ayer products. As well as claiming Madame Récamier, Mrs Ayer approached celebrated contemporary women and asked them to endorse her cream. Her first 'name' was Adelina Patti.

Another advocate was Lily Langtry, the English society beauty.

It could have been suggested that the Jersey Lily would endorse anything for money; and Pears' soap had paid her £150 for a famous series of advertisements. As a child of fourteen Lily's beauty had been suspect in her own home where the villagers suggested that she covered her face with minced raw meat at night to sustain her youthful complexion, and that her alabaster skin was acquired by rolling naked in the dew. These expedients showed a profit, for when she was twenty-four, this pale, violet-eyed girl made her entrance into London society on the arm of her reputedly rich husband. Her first appearance, at a dinner party, caused a sensation and in the same week Lord Randolph Churchill wrote to his wife: 'I dined with Lord Wharncliffe last night and took into dinner a Mrs Langtry, a most beautiful creature quite unknown, very poor, and they say has but one black dress'. This was May 1877, and that one black dress, worn in mourning for her brother, sustained Mrs Langtry for so many social engagements that when Lady Dudley invited her to a ball she asked the girl to wear something different. The white velvet dress which replaced it caused such a furore that the guests stood on chairs to see Lily Langtry pass. After this adventure she was to be mobbed in the streets; her face appeared on picture cards, in portraits for the Academy, and in a pencil sketch above the bed of Prince Leopold. It was removed by his mother, and the indignant Queen Victoria mounted a chair to do so.

It is doubtful if Lily Langtry needed cosmetics in the early years of her career as a professional beauty. She had to be instructed by Mrs Labouchère in the necessity to dab cold cream behind her lower lip when she made her first stage appearance. This was to stop her from biting her lips with terror.

By 1882 Mrs Langtry was more sophisticated. She was celebrated as the mistress of the Prince of Wales and had engaged in a theatrical career which had resulted in enormous success although the critics felt this was rather owing to her notoriety than to her acting ability. She was a professional beauty, her

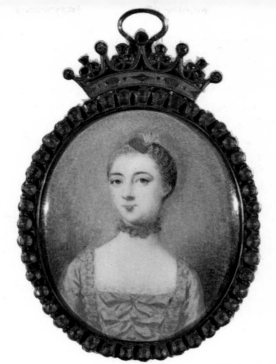

Penelope Cotes *Maria Gunning, Countess of Coventry* 1757. Wallace Collection, London
The most famous 'victim to Cosmetics'

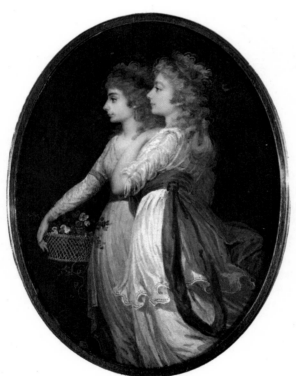

P. N. Guérin *Georgiana, Duchess of Devonshire and Lady Elizabeth Foster c.* 1791. Wallace
Collection, London
Their hoydenish prettiness contrasts with the stiff beauty of the earlier ideal
represented by Maria Gunning.

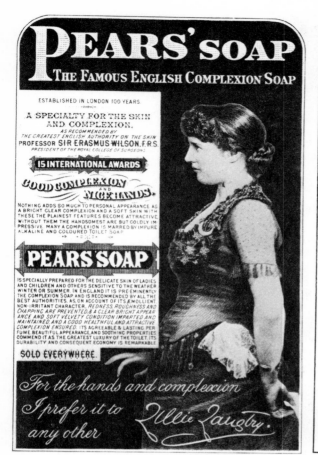

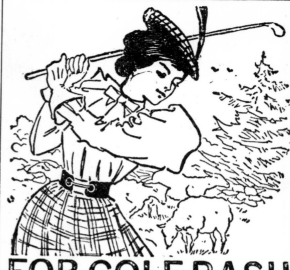

FOR GOLF RASH

Heat Rash, inflammation, itching, irritation, and chafing, undue or offensive perspiration, and many sanative uses, nothing is so cooling, purifying, and refreshing as a bath with CUTICURA SOAP, greatest of skin beautifiers and purest of toilet soaps, and gentle anointings with CUTICURA, purest of emollient skin cures.

Sold everywhere. British depot: F. NEWBERY & SONS London. French depot: L. MIDY, Paris. Australian depot: R. TOWNS & Co., Sydney. POTTER DRUG AND CHEM. CORP., Sole Props., Boston, U. S. A.

Left Advertisement for Pears', 1890s. Lily Langtry

Right Advertisement for Cuticura, 1890s. The 'New Woman'

clothes were simple dresses by Worth, chosen to show her tall, rather plump figure and her white shoulders. Her jewellery, culled from some of the richest men in England and America, was elaborate and famous, including a stomacher formerly worn by the Empress Eugénie. During her tour of America, a Boston reporter visited her dressing-room and described it:

Her dressing-table is of white wood, heavily enamelled in white, the table is elaborately mounted with cupids and butterflies, delicately made and fringed with old rose satin with muslin beneath peeping through at the top. The mirror is electrically lighted to Mrs Langtry's own special design and by an ingenious colour arrangement colour effects, blue, red, and amber can be obtained at will . . . For the reception of the very numerous articles of toilette there is a sort of tray. Nearly everything on this table is of gold. Each brush, comb, scent bottle, powder box and the like is engraved with Mrs Langtry's initials.

One can imagine the earnest reporter, stub of licked pencil in hand, making hasty notes on his pad before the actress came to greet him. She did not like reporters and when she visited Armour's the Chicago slaughterhouse she compared a scaly red bristled pig with a newspaperman.

Her boxes and powder could be displayed in a theatre dressing room for actresses needed these artificial aids, but when she furnished her own home at Regal Lodge in Ascot there was no sign of cosmetics. Her elegant bedroom was sumptuous, even the shower was silver plated, and she had two dressing tables, one of which displayed the brushes and combs of the Prince of Wales. The bed-cover was purple and gold with E.R. and a crown blazoned on it in gold, but in the centre of this flagrant exhibition of her power, Mrs Langtry's own dressing table was empty of any lotions or cosmetic boxes.

By 1900 the Jersey Lily was wilting; after an appearance in New York an observer said 'the whitewash with which she was covered did not conceal the hollows and wrinkles and roughness.' Kinder critics said that she still had a Grecian perfection, although she was now termed handsome rather than beautiful. When she was asked her beauty secrets she said she had 'learnt to keep my thoughts young'.

In 1890 a remarkable fashion suggested that the world of the demi-monde had fused with that of the respectable woman. For the latest cosmetic art was breast piercing. The nipples were lacerated in order to wear gold or jewelled pins. A letter to a magazine says:

For a long time I could not understand why I should consent to such a painful operation without sufficient reason. I soon however came to the conclusion that many ladies are prepared to bear passing pain for the sake of love. I found that the breasts of the ladies who wore rings were incomparably rounder and fuller developed than those who did not . . . so I had my nipples pierced and when the wounds were healed I had rings inserted . . . I can only say they are not in the least uncomfortable or painful. On the contrary, the slight rubbing and slipping of the rings causes in me a titillating feeling . . .

Since the 'eighties it had been a current complaint that young ladies had no sense of morality. Their outdoor sports, their bloomers and their slang had sent more than one elder lady reaching for her sal volatile. The fashionable beauty had changed. In England the Pre-Raphaelites had introduced a new conception: Mrs H. R. Haweis wrote in *The Art of Beauty* in 1878:

Morris, Burne Jones and others have made certain types of face and figure, once literally hated, actually the fashion. Red hair—once to say a woman had red hair was social assassination—is all the rage. A pallid face with a protruding upper lip is highly esteemed. Green eyes, a squint, square eyebrows, whitey-brown complexions are not left out in the cold. Now is the time for plain women.

There ensued a direct conflict between the New Woman and femininity. The New Woman, slightly lesbian, would smoke cigarettes and lounge about on the sofa. She swaggered in check suits and hard pork-pie hats. Her mode was a contradiction with the beauties celebrated by society painters, whose décolleté necklines might have held two or three Maréchal Niel roses and whose bodies were fragrant with violets or heliotrope. They were often fragrant with other smells: an elderly lady noticing the twentieth-century preoccupation with deodorants mentioned that at the turn of the century men liked to smell a little sweat 'we called it *bouquet de corsage*'.

In 1895 the well-known Ada Leverson was wearing applied make-up. As a novelist she was allowed more latitude than society hostesses, but her more

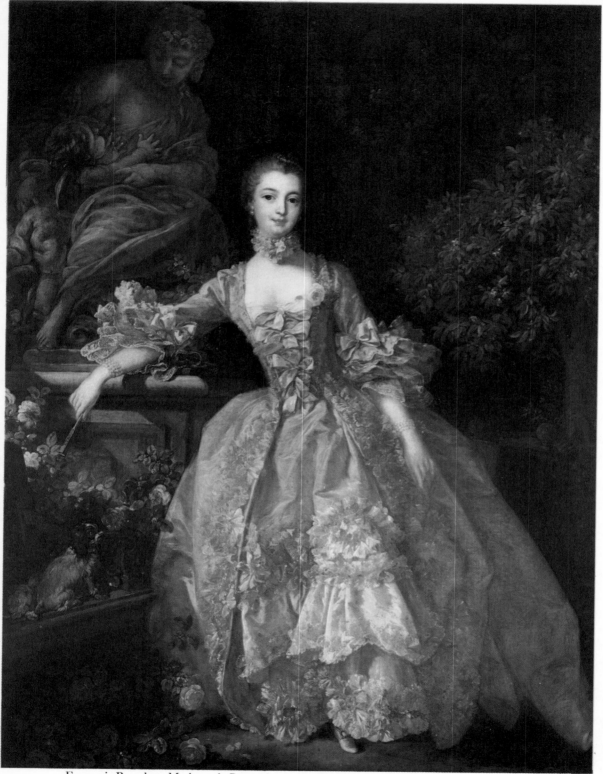

François Boucher *Madame de Pompadour* 1759. Wallace Collection, London
The faint sheen on her skin suggests the presence of cosmetics, an impression French
portrait painters, unlike their English counterparts, were quite happy to give.

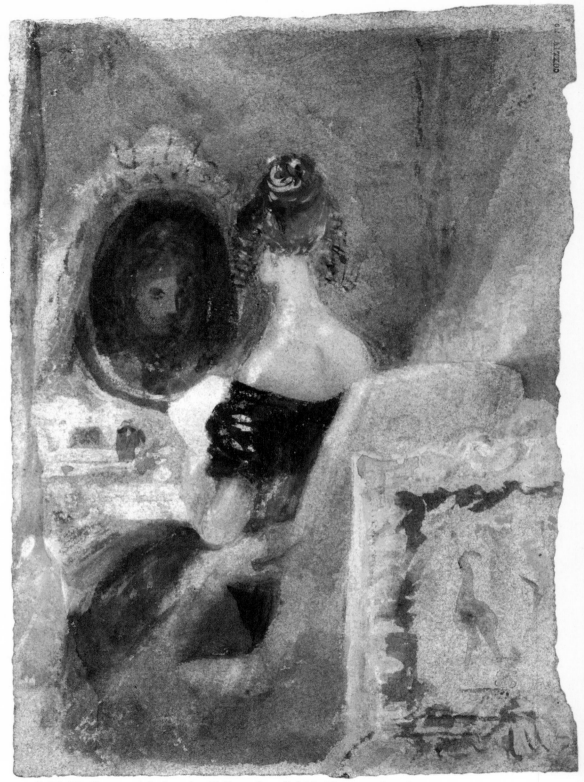

J. M. W. Turner *A Lady at her Toilette* 1830. British Museum, London
The early-nineteenth-century dressing table as seen by Turner

105

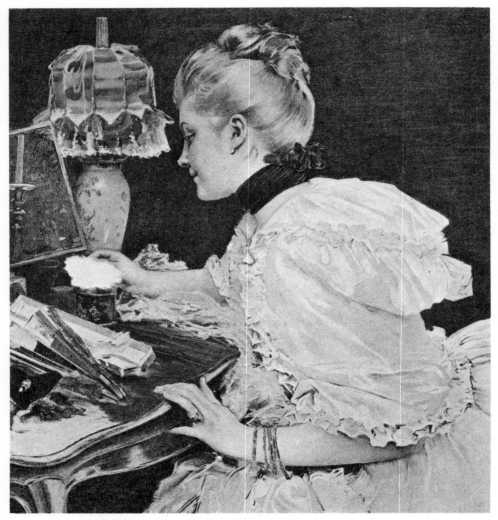

Preparing for the Ball engraving after L. Doucet, 1891
The touch of powder has survived the nineteenth-century morality, and perhaps
this French woman has deserted rice powder for the more cunning notions of the new
cosmeticians. Her lip salve and rouge are concealed, only a demi-mondaine or an
actress would display them on her dressing table.

rigidly conventional husband objected strongly to her cosmetics and her
daughter remembers: 'Often when dressed to go out to dinner together the
Sphinx would be sent back to her room in tears to scrub her face from suspected
rouge.' Men might be permitted to use unguents. The same perceptive little
girl would wait in the hall of the house at 19 Hyde Park Place to smell the top
hats of gentlemen visitors which were redolent with the smell of hair oil. She
adds: 'Scent was much used by dandies on their hair and by women of bad

reputation. Ladies seldom wore anything stronger than lavender water or that rather mysterious and unpleasant scent known as orris root.'

Mrs Leverson persisted with her cosmetics, perhaps feeling that her adherence to Oscar Wilde had already sent her beyond the boundaries of more pallid Victorian Society. In 1906 Marcel Boulestin met her in Paris and accused her of peroxiding her hair. She said that she merely darkened a little at the roots. In the 'twenties, Osbert Sitwell noticed how brilliant her lips were, and how golden her hair. The young girls of the 'eighties and 'nineties enjoyed defying convention. They began to redden their lips and paint their cheeks, occasioning Max Beerbohm's essay 'On the Pervasion of Rouge' and this swan song for the simple Victorian heroine:

The Victorian era comes to an end and the day of sancta simplicitas is quite ended. The old signs are here and the portents to warn the seer of life that we are ripe for a new age of artifice. Are not men rattling the dice box and ladies dipping their fingers in the rouge pots? Last century too, when life was lived by candlelight and ethics was but etiquette and even art a question of punctilio, women, we know, gave the best hours of the day to the crafty farding of their faces and the towering of their coiffures.

The young dandy continued that it was curious that a prejudice existed against cosmetics so that 'all things were sacrificed to the fetish Nature'. In an age when the queen's face was enamelled he could add that 'artifice's first command to them is that they should repose. With bodily activity their powder will fly, their enamel crack'. With nostalgia he remembers the unpainted actress, Cissie Loftus, who was 'like a daisy in the window of Solomon's'.

It was true that Mrs Frances Henning had a back door to her salon. This business in South Molton Street sold creams and lotions as well as three shades of rouge. Her customers came up to the first floor where the cunning Mrs Henning would interview them in quiet closed rooms. A negro maid stood at the turn of the stairs, watching to see that privacy was respected. The grooms and horsey gentlemen who strolled in the mews behind must have imagined that the salon was a high-class house of assignation as the veiled ladies passed through the alley, swaying on the cobblestones and avoiding the steaming piles of dung. The salon flourished and became the house of Cyclax.

But Mrs Henning's business would not have succeeded ten years earlier, or in a lower social stratum. The middle- and upper-class women had to preserve the myth that she was natural. The grander aristocracy could flagrantly wear make-up. Queen Alexandra's enamelled face shocked and amused close observers, but the population tacitly ignored her maquillage of white and red.

Magazines of the 'nineties were discreetly advertising cosmetics. At the time when Harriet Hubbard Ayer entered journalism, 'puffs' were appearing in this country which were less subtle than her stories of Mme Récamier. They included 'Crème Admiratrice, the only preparation for restoring the clear and healthy appearance of a youthful complexion; Veloutine powder; eyebrow pencils; Fard Indien in all shades for darkening and improving the eyebrows; Bâton au Raisin for the lips.' The tight corseting at the end of the century accentuated the aggravating 'green sickness' which was identified as chlorosis.

However the renewed acceptance of cosmetics was to create a market for those branded creams which were the forerunners of present day cosmetics.

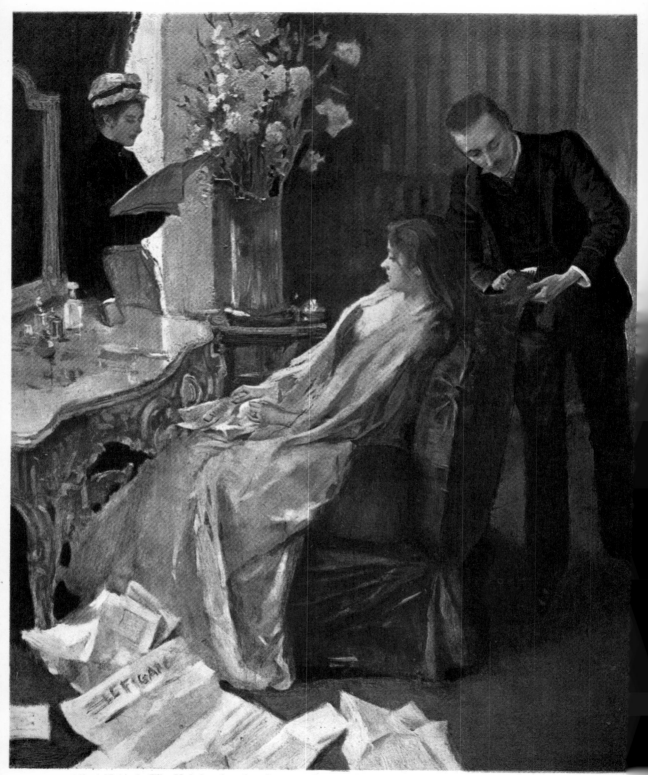

Albert Lynch *The Hairdressing Appointment* 1891
Fashionable ladies had their hair done in absolute privacy by a visiting hairdresser.

In the 1890s young Helena Rubinstein emigrated from Poland to Australia: 'As the date of my departure neared, I packed my old-fashioned trunk with all my possessions, including twelve pots of my mother's beauty cream,' she recollected in her autobiography. This cream had been recommended by a visiting actress, who had commissioned it from a chemist, Dr Jacob Lykusky. It contained herbs and essence of almonds. When Helena Rubinstein arrived in her new home: 'My friends could not get over the texture and milkiness of my skin. It was in fact no better than the average girl's in my home town in Poland, but to the ladies of Victoria, with their sun-scorched, wind-burned cheeks, the city-bred alabaster quality seemed remarkable.' She sent home for twelve pots for her friends and as demands for the cream increased, the young girl asked for more and more pots which she stored in the cellar to maintain them at the right temperature. Finally, she borrowed £250 and opened a beauty salon. She invited Dr Lykusky to join her and began to compound varying creams for different skin types. There was still prejudice against the use of colour and the early Rubinstein products, like those of Harriet Hubbard Ayer, were concentrated on medicated uses.

The famous name still sold cream. The advertisement of Miss Nellie Steward established the Rubinstein product. She was an English actress who found that the Australian climate affected her skin, and who brought her friend Nellie Melba to the salon. 'It was then about 1908. Make-up was used exclusively for stage purposes and actresses were the only women who knew anything of the art, or who would dare to be seen in public wearing anything but the lightest film of rice powder.'

This dread rice powder had supplanted ceruse as the artificial whitener of the skin. It came from China and not only made the face appear whitewashed, but it would swell in the pores of the skin and enlarge them. Its livid appearance made make-up immediately obvious and Helena Rubinstein realized that a tinted face powder would not only seem more natural, but that this would recommend it to a larger public. Colour was still virtually unknown in spite of the red lips of the hoydenish girls of the 'nineties. But one person who appreciated the use of camouflage was Gabrielle Ray, an actress who showed Helena Rubinstein how to shade the skin at the corners of her nostrils with red or mauve dots which reduced the size of the nose. She also put a little shadow on her eyes and over the temples 'to enhance the size and luminosity of her eyes'. With a hare's foot she dabbed colour over her cheeks, the lobes of her ears and her chin. When Helena Rubinstein opened her salon in London she did not have to wait for customers. They came veiled, and no lady carried money with her. But they were prepared to pay considerable sums.

In Paris it was the age of the Belle Epoque. Those fragile years between the turn of the century and the first world war were pervaded with the colour and scents of the high-class courtesans as well as the fashionable ladies who made France seem filled with feminine enchantment. Yet in spite of those extravagant ladies like Emilie d'Alençon and La Belle Otéro, there was a curious ignorance about the application of cosmetics. The French seemed to be waiting for an outsider to aid them. In 1901 an American cosmetician, Mrs Anna Ruppert, advertised that she was coming to Paris and bringing with her 'a beautiful complexion . . . [which] is within the reach of almost all, and can be acquired by nearly every woman who will take the trouble to look after her skin'.

14 The Edwardian beauty salon

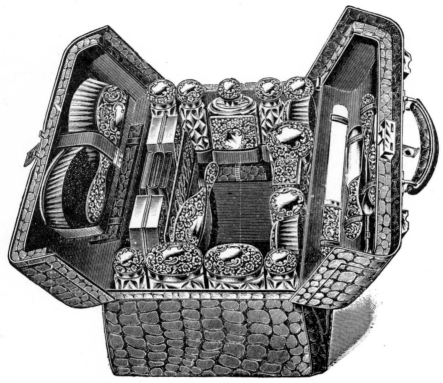

Mappin & Webb dressing case, 1897
'"Engadine" Dressing Bag in Real Crocodile, completely fitted with Chased
Sterling Silver and Richly Cut Glass Toilet Requisites.'

It is ironic that in spite of the strictures of the Victorian moralists the complexion
of the virtuous woman at the end of the period was ravaged rather than radiant.
The heavy diet filled with carbohydrates, the lack of exercise and fresh air,
combined with a determination not to ease the problems of dry skin and dirt,
made the late Victorian lady an unalluring sight.

One historian claims that it was the only period when women attempted
to gain attention by looking older than their years, for they pushed their
figures into the heavy S-shape which would be celebrated by Charles Gibson's
drawings at the turn of the century. One of the most famous beauties of 1902
was Camille Clifford, a young girl who contrived with the aid of corsetry,
black velvet, and a horsehair pad under her own hair, to look like a dowager
in late middle age. One theory, which seems logical, is that the ideal of the
age was the type of woman who appealed to the Prince of Wales, now in late

Edwardian ladies became objects of adoration to their children, who always seemed
to remember them as sweet smelling, exquisitely dressed and elegant. Later, memoir
writers mourned the passing of their sense of style with the first world war.

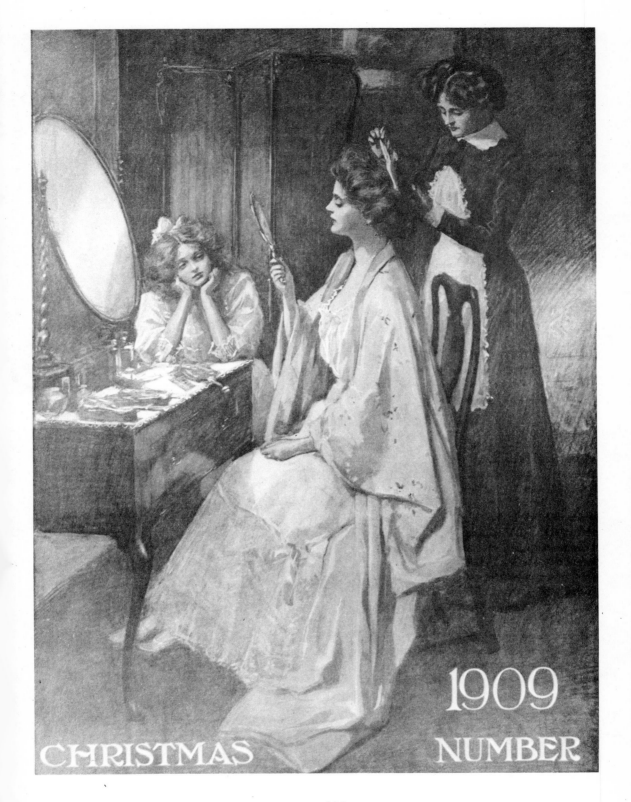

1909

CHRISTMAS NUMBER

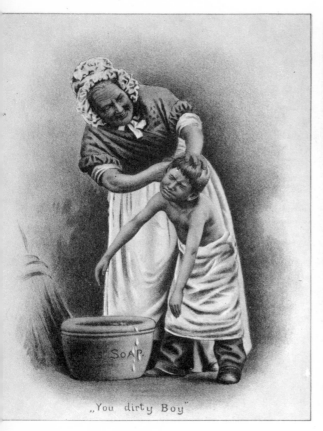

"You dirty Boy"

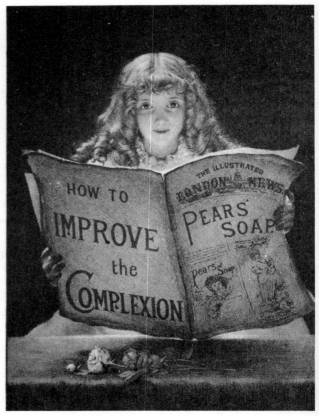

Cover of booklet advertising Pears' soap, 1890s
The advertisements for Pears' soap were the forerunners of the propaganda concerned with purity and child-like complexions.

middle age himself, and so youth was discarded at the age of sixteen so that the lady in society might appear as a heavy, dominating creature escaped from a Du Maurier cartoon.

These lethargic goddess figures overcast the late Victorian and Edwardian age, completely in command of their own lives and the affairs of all about them. It was a matriarchal system . . . the poems about 'mother' proliferated in a period when so many men disappeared to the Empire and conjured up their homes with sentimental ditties addressed to those women, like the old queen, who were infuriatingly more important than their wives. The extreme poise of the Edwardian upper-class woman in middle age is admirably described in a short paragraph by Sonia Keppel recalling her mother, Alice Keppel, whose beauty had captivated the elderly Prince of Wales. At the turn of the century she accompanied her mother on a railway journey during which they slept in wagons-lits:

Throughout her life Mamma wore her beauty without vanity as she would an old mackintosh. Now, aesthetically, acutely I minded the way she obliterated it for the night. Out of a square silk case she brought a small pillow, a shapeless nightgown and a mob cap. Under the nightgown she subdued her beautifully curved body. And under the cap, she piled her shining chestnut hair. Next she greased her face. Then she helped me up the ladder to my upper berth and kissed me 'good-night'.

This incongruous picture is of one of the most sophisticated Edwardians, for most of them were afraid to pamper their skins and bodies. Supplementary teeth and hair were all the lower income groups could admit. Baths were not encouraged, even the country-house gentry would think twice about the problems of carrying jugs of hot water along endless corridors to add to a lukewarm tub. Most people still washed sparsely in cold water, and as the ladies wore veils perhaps their skins were not seen too clearly.

'Face enamelling' gained some acceptance among the rich after 1900, perhaps because of the revelation of Alexandra. Rouge was still considered the prerogative of the demi-monde, although many of the most exquisite examples of high-stepping 'pretty horse-breakers' of the Victorian age had been renowned for their charming natural complexions.

Although they had been termed the 'highly tinted Venuses' by a writer in the *Saturday Review*, the rich courtesans had become a pleasant myth in English society. The later Victorian moralists had been disturbed by the fact that chaste young ladies might sigh away over the heroine of *La Traviata*, and that the most accomplished of the loose young ladies were received everywhere except in court circles, as if they were actually an asset to their society.

A world in which an elderly or middle-aged man could marry a young debutante, while a younger man was not eligible owing to lack of money entailed that many businessmen and aristocrats had to beguile their time with the 'Skittles', 'Laura Bells' and 'Agnes Willoughbys', who plied their hire by riding in the Row.

The respectable woman was not immune to the blandishments of cosmetics. *Papier poudré* was a resort which whitened their blue noses in winter, and their shining cheeks in the summer. It came in small books containing leaves of coloured paper, which were pressed against the cheeks; and they used burnt matchsticks to darken their eyelashes. Like the ladies of earlier centuries they utilized geranium and poppy petals to stain their lips.

Most 'nice' women used Pears' soap, which had amazing sales at the turn of the century, accelerated by clever advertising.

Many manufactureres of household remedies were aware of the potential in cosmetics. Chesebrough-Ponds, makers of Vaseline and vetinary extracts for cattle, realized at the end of the nineteenth century that their chemical knowledge might be put to profitable use in the face creams and lotions.

Vaseline was advertised on the sides of horsebuses and trolleys, it had become a term which many people did not appreciate was a brand name, and Edwardian ladies experimented with it to shine their chapped lips. It was used as a base for hair tonic, soap, harness oil and axle grease. In 1905 Ponds enlarged their scope to more cosmetic matters, still insisting that their products were medicinal rather than attractive. This litany had to be repeated by many manufacturers of the time, who could not claim that they were aiding the general impetus towards immorality. Pond's Extract was mysteriously used for Constipation, Cold in the Head, Hay Fever, Malarial Fever, Syphilis and Typhoid Fever, according to a popular booklet of 1905 in which Toilet Articles were expected to go unnoticed among the general medicinal qualities. The Americans were less prudish. A year before Harriet Hubbard Ayer had written a booklet for the Pond's Extract Company, called *Beauty, A Woman's Birthright* and subtitled *How Every Woman May Look Her Best*. It was an inspiration, for it appeared at a

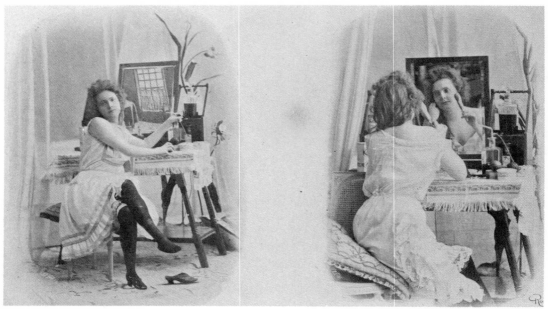

Advertisement for Lenthéric, 1890s
Lenthéric used audacious photographs in this advertisement.

time when most women were hoping for some arguments to support their desire for cosmetics, and Mrs Ayer's opening paragraph defined the general attitude in the United States: 'The time has gone by, fortunately, when it was regarded as sinful for a woman to take the same tender care of herself and her appearance as she piously bestowed on the parlour furniture and the dining-room silverware.' In spite of this preliminary note the book continues to stress the healing properties of Pond's Extract Cream rather than its cosmetic advantages. However, she did give detailed instructions for a 'Cream Bath'.

Although this suggests that attitudes were slightly altered many women who had succumbed to the theory of cosmetics were indecisive about choosing a brand. Memories remained of the notorious Madame Rachel who had opened a shop in Bond Street in the 1860s where she sold highly priced toilet waters and, under the counter, tinted face powder. Madame Rachel was in a splendid position to blackmail and dupe her clients and her career had ended with a sentence to five years' imprisonment after she had gained all the wealth of a Mrs Borrodale who had bought every creation of the House of Rachel until she was completely in the power of the adventuress. Madame Rachel was sentenced as Mrs Sarah Rachel Leverson, and the duplicity of the creators of the smart salon and beauty preparations had created suspicion in the minds of a later potential public.

They were more easily persuaded by those toilet preparations issued by old-established manufacturers, even if they were less exciting than those which arrived from the continent or which contained tints and perfumes. Large soap manufacturers such as Yardley had been favourites with a small middle-class public since the Great Exhibition in 1851, and they had even more chance of success with the toilet waters which they introduced in the early 1900s. This decision also signalled the growing importance of a brand name, for although the name of Yardley and Co. was recognised by people in the trade, most of their twopenny bars of soap had been retailed under the names of the individual chemists. In the nineteenth century, people in a small community felt that it was safer to buy the supposed locally made product from a family shop, with which they had dealt for generations, but as the new skill of advertising grew, the large organisation with nation-wide application was to replace the family store. Yardley appreciated this at the point when public attitudes were altering, and so they were able to establish a reputation which appealed to two facets of the British public taste. They were an old firm (established in 1770), and so they had the charm of authenticity and respect within the trade; and at the same time they appealed to the public which wanted a well-known name on a product which might be bought in every chemist's in the country and which would have the same quality everywhere. They also appealed to sentiment with their use of a package design incorporating Wheatley's engraving of a primrose seller from the 'Cries of London' series. The primrose seller, used for the first time in 1919, was skilfully altered to a lavender pedlar . . . for lavender was, even at that late date, redolent with nostalgia for high quality and ladylike attributes.

Lavender water or a refined cologne was the only admissible perfume for a lady before the first world war. Sachets were tucked into breasts and layers of sheets, and most households made up their own lavender bags, even if they bought manufactured perfume. Only the poorest girls or a fast woman used Phul-Nana which was cheap, and which appeared in a highly coloured package; another 'servant girls' scent' was called Shem-el Nessim, which must have caused much tongue twisting when it was bought in the penny bazaars . . . Every woman over a certain age curled her hair with tight curlers made by Hindes, or else with lethal looking iron tongs.

The colours of dresses reflected the feeling for lavender smells; Cecil Beaton remembered that Edwardian ladies of his circle under a certain age wore sweet-pea colours 'so their make-up was of a restricted palette; lips were touched with coral, instead of carmine, complexions were peaches and cream. Hair was pale nut brown and I remember that the yellow or peroxide hair which we now call blonde, was at the time considered unfortunate.' An interesting piece of extra information reveals that women had little use for handbags. Although middle-aged ladies carried reticules which might contain knitting there was evidently no parallel to the complex mixture of cigarettes, cheque books, cosmetics and purses which we know today, for Anthony Glyn remarks: 'Evening bags were never used, as cosmetics were at that time almost unknown in society circles, and could only be bought at theatrical costumiers'.'

Ironically, the French looked to England for advice on beauty, although this situation would be altered after the war. London beauticians invaded Paris in 1909. The most popular were Mrs and Miss Earle who came by the unlikely route of Liverpool and Manchester to 279 rue St Honoré, to establish the English Institute of Beauty. After their successes in the north country they could claim to 'restore freshness to faded faces' and they found a ready public, for in the same year the fashion journal of France, *Les Modes,* had included a stern dissertation to its readers: 'It is for her complexion above all that a woman should worry. Its beauty is not easy to maintain, for the diaphanous pellicule which is the top layer of skin is of extreme delicacy.'

The sensitive attitude to colour was dispelled rudely by the arrival in Paris of the Russian Ballet in 1910. (See page 132.) It is almost impossible to estimate now the effect this theatrical troupe had on western European fashions. Many women who had their cosmetics and clothes irretrievably altered by the hectic

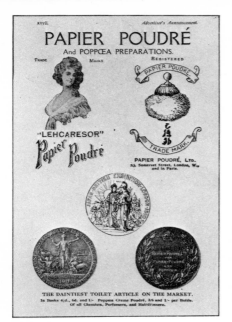

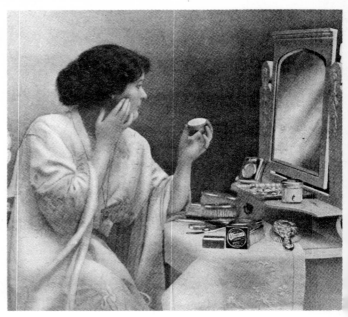

Left From the *Daily Mirror Beauty Book* 1910
Papier poudré came in the form of a booklet and the torn-out pages were applied to
one's cheeks.
Right Advertisement for Vinolia, 1913
By 1913 cosmetics could be displayed on the dressing table, but the creams were
still intended to act as preservatives, not to add colour.

designs of Poiret, could hardly have appreciated that the colour was inaugurated by a theatrical trick. Bright colours had been inadmissible for over a
century. The most distinctive shades were the heavy ochres and crimsons
which were acceptable wear for wives of opulent Victorian manufacturers.
One could almost say that lively colour had been banished with the French
Revolution, and that it took a miniature Russian revolution of taste to establish
it again. The reintroduction of brilliant shades began, of course, with a few
women who had audacity and high incomes. One very good reason for dull
dress in the lower income groups was that clothes had to last in an age when
there was no dry cleaning . . . therefore black, navy and grey were the expected
colours for an elderly woman to wear; and young girls might use paler shades
only if they were in washable materials. Cecil Beaton's view of sweet-pea shades
was of a restricted society in which dresses could be discarded. Yet even then a
dress could not be too obtrusive. An earlier generation had been hypnotized
by Lily Langtry's white velvet dress because it was so impractical. Yet the
Edwardians took to the colours of the Russian Ballet with the same abandon
as they took to the American barn dance.

The Daily Mirror Beauty Book, published in 1910, reflected the fact that for
the literate classes, cosmetics were acceptable; However, much of their advice
still incorporates home-made lotions: the manufactured ones might still be
considered spurious:

LIP ROUGE

Boric Acid	3 drachms
Carmine	$\frac{1}{4}$ drachm
Soft Paraffin	2 ounces
Hard Paraffin	1 ounce

Otto of Rose, sufficient to perfume.

This avant-garde little booklet also suggested a pencil line to elongate the eyes; devices to make the eyelashes turn upwards and make them 'look like stars'; a home-made eyebrow darkener created from gum arabic, Indian ink and rosewater; and astringent lotion. The advertisements were also revolutionary, including one for the 'Veedee', which was a vibrator and which seemed to be a panacea for baldness, double chins, poor complexions, wrinkles, pallor, fatness and thinness . . . it was accompanied by a reference from Lily Langtry, as well as the names of fifteen other enthusiasts, with a wide range of titles.

Some of the aristocracy found a novel way to make up. George Burchett was a famous tattooist in an age when the tattoo reached immense popularity in Britain. In 1910 many people had 'Coronation tattoos' done, showing the royal arms or a patriotic motto; and even Lady Randolph Churchill was decorated.

George Burchett was practising at a time when many women were hesitant about cosmetics. They were still restricted to the aristocracy or the very rich who might patronize the young Miss Rubinstein's salon. However electrolysis had been accepted as a method to remove hair, and it was obvious that if the practice of make-up were to extend to the lower orders, the upper classes would need similar novelties to sustain them in their search for beauty.

Burchett was approached by a Monsieur de Barri, who had opened a salon at 17 North Audley Street, with a Doctor A.W. Wheatley. Burchett called two or three times a week to aid those 'Dainty Tints Imprinted on Society Ladies' Cheeks'. Pink blushes, red lips and dark eyebrows were needled in, although the word tattoo was never mentioned, and harmless vegetable matter was injected just under the skin to give a natural look. From this salon, Burchett moved to that of 'Kosmos' at 80 Duke Street, which was in a house shared with Madame Josephine, the court dressmaker. Kosmos was a product of his profession and period, in his early thirties with a waxed moustache and a self-employed reference, as 'the only beauty specialist with seven years' practical experience in leading European hospitals'. He advertised treatment for:

Superfluous hair; Moles, Warts; Discoloration; Treatments of Troubles in the Veins; Corrections of Malformed Noses; Prominent Ears; Special Treatment for Bust Development and a Patented Method for the Treatment of Obesity and Slenderness.

Carefully the word 'tattoo' was released at a point when it would become a rage rather than a slur; and the volume of trade increased amazingly, for the tattoo had become a fashionable idiosyncrasy which everybody wished to have; Burchett's card stated that he would perform cosmetic miracles:

> Complexions permanently tinted
> Eyes shaded—Lips shaded and coloured
> Scars tinted—Noses whitened.
> Moles, Blemishes and Tattoo marks removed

and of course, replaced with another, more subtle, tattooed complexion.

This seemingly crude beauty treatment was to be used to great effect in a grimmer cause, for George Burchett turned to tattooing the men disfigured by the first world war, inserting skin tones in battered faces, and covering

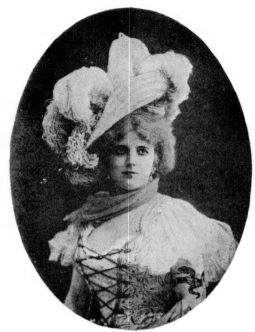

The Princess Chimay, who was tattooed on her arms, cheeks and lips in Cairo in 1899
Tattooing became a method of gaining a permanently pink complexion; some
fashionable women carried the practice to extremes.

scars with more sightly colours.

The swan song of the era was not the death of Edward VII. He succumbed to cosmetics at the end, for Willie Clarkson, the theatrical costumier and make-up artist, was asked to insert colour into the cheeks of the dying king. This remedy had been used earlier by another ruler, for Napoleon III had rouged his cheeks before the Battle of Sedan in the Franco-Prussian War of 1870, anxious that the ravages of dysentery and worry should not be too apparent to his disconsolate men.

So the old king passed, made up to his former ruddy self; but the real aubade to his era came four years later, although the *Gazette du Bon Ton* could hardly have appreciated it when they accepted a piece by the Comte de Fleury, which was aptly described by James Laver, in *Edwardian Promenade*, as the perfect picture of Paris before its twentieth-century deluge:

In the motor cars, the coupés, one sees enveloped in lace, tulle, light satins, full of reflections. ladies of all ages but chiefly in the summer of life, the full flowering of their youth, like roses garnishing the dinner table, and who also have their drops of water, the tears of their coronets and necklaces on the flesh of their shoulders and the curls of their hair . . . . It is dinner time, dinner time in summer, the heat of the day is over. The heavens turn green and the last rays of the sun lend an orange tint to the sky which hangs like a velarium over the Bois de Bologne.

It was the warm summer of 1914.

15 The mass market

The exclusive male franchise was not the only victim of the first world war. With the growing emancipation of women came an equal emancipation in their dress and attitudes, for the girls who had their hair bobbed to avoid machinery in the munitions factories, or to keep it out of their eyes as they nursed wounded soldiers, were hardly capable of turning back to ankle-length skirts and the heavy chignons which had been in favour before the war; the holocaust very much accelerated a process which had begun before the war.

It was generally accepted that women were flighty before 1914; the Jazz Age had begun, and was postponed rather than inaugurated by the war. The factor which determined the growing acceptance of cosmetics was, initially, the cinema. Nudes, of a restrained, plump, and furtive type, were shown on the screen in 1918; they presaged a liberation which would ironically turn back upon itself, as censorship entered the American movie industry. However, the cosmetics of Theda Bara caused a minor revolution in make-up; she was portrayed, her real face heavily disguised, by Helena Rubinstein. This pioneer in the cosmetic industry had gone to New York after her success in Britain and Australia. Her innovations had included the use of coloured powder, and she had grasped the ideas of colour-shaded eyes from the French stage. She created mascara for Theda Bara, relying heavily on her experiments with kohl; and the heavy-lidded eyes, bland white face and carefully reddened mouth gave cinema audiences in Britain and America a new view of femininity.

Another aspect of the increasing growth of interest in cosmetics was caused by a completely new consideration of marriage. Until the 'twenties women could only be emancipated by marriage, and then only with their husbands' approval. A few women of the upper classes, with money of their own, might be able to break away from the drawing room tedium, but only if they were in revolutionary households. Even in a family like the Darwins, one of the most scholarly and progressive of the late nineteenth century, there was a retinue of aunts, who might be fortunate enough to live alone, or rather with a companion; but who would travel accompanied, and whose cosmetic ideals began and ended with brown oatmeal soap. As the numbers of eligible men dwindled rapidly with deaths in the war, women gained new confidence. It was true that many of them could not hope to marry, there were not enough men to go round, but in the absence of men during the war, they had increasingly taken men's jobs; or those which had been regarded as male provinces before 1914. The hurly-burly of the war determined that even the most gentle-born woman had to jostle on buses, travel alone by train, and also meet contemporary problems and have to make decisions which would never have been presented to her before.

Accepting their position as 'bachelor girls' many women set up flats, apart from the families with whom they would have lived before (even to death) to preserve their gentility. The emancipated middle-class girl was a freak at first considered by some commentators to be a lesbian, owing to the intense relationships which occurred at a time when men were scarce and women had to attempt new work, new methods of living and new characterizations. They

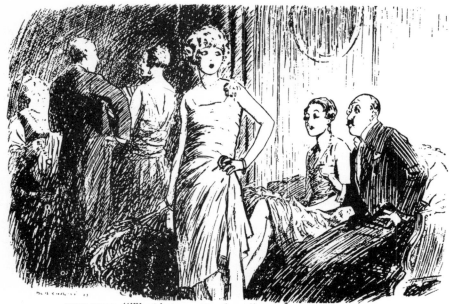

THE MAN. "That's a pretty face."
THE WOMAN. "Yes—but they're not being worn like that."

A cartoon of the 'twenties reproduced in *Mr Punch in Mayfair* published 1933

also had money which they had earned—not inherited—and with this they could buy the cosmetics which were beginning to flood the market. Many of the manufacturers of the present day were established during the 'twenties and 'thirties, and their domination began in a period when there was a clamour for new types of cosmetics. A working girl might now buy cosmetics for the first time. She had made her own, somewhat inadequately, in the past, and as she began to rouge and use lipstick, there was an appreciable outcry from her employers. Women who attempted extreme forms of make-up for themselves could not accept it in their general servants, or in shop assistants. It was a typical moral criticism of the period; and many girls were sacked because they tinted their lips audaciously, in spite of the class system which pertained against it. The new trends occasioned another ironic reversal of class badges, for while the over-cosmeticized woman of the 'twenties was almost always of the upper income groups, the similar woman of the 'thirties, and after, was almost certainly identifiable as a worker. One can hypothesize on the reasons; that the servant imitated the aristocrat; that the unemployed of the later years needed make-up to bring some colour into their unnaturally anxious and drab lives; or simply that cosmetics became cheaper.

They certainly reached everybody's handbag. It is sad that many young working women of the inter-war years did much better, financially, than most men; they were employed readily for their labour was comparatively cheap and they generally had no dependants. All they earned was for pleasure after the rent had been paid, and cheaper cosmetics had large sales. The psychology of the lipstick, known to every woman today, was initiated at this time. A miserable woman received some relief from her sorrow in spending money. Usually a new dress was too expensive, even in the 'twenties, so she bought a lipstick instead; whether it was the phallic significance of the article, or simply that it was the most colourful cheap cosmetic, lipsticks sold and sold in a way which was unattainable by rouge or powder. Forty years later, this phenomenon was even more significant.

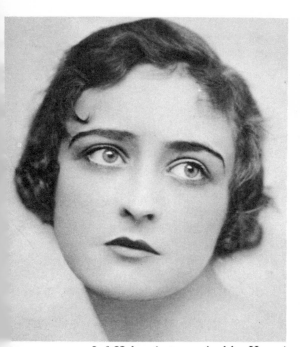 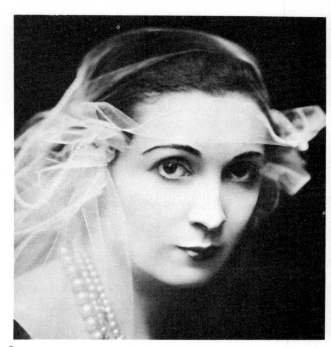

Left Hebe photographed by Hoppé, 1928
Hebe was a famous model and her face was an English ideal of the 'twenties,
yet it recalls some of the softness of the black-stockinged girls of the Edwardian age
who put their hair up when they were seventeen.

Right Lady Lavery photographed by Hoppé, 1925
Lady Lavery's natural beauty was a forecast of the deceptive fragility and uncos-
meticized fashion of the 'sixties; an unkind critic said that the admiral who inaugurated
camouflage did so after a dinner party where he sat opposite Lady Lavery.

The great decision of the 'twenties was whether to bob hair; it was a change
whose significance it is now difficult to convey; it typified the onset of a new
personality in a period when one was labelled according to whether hair was
bobbed or not. Scott Fitzgerald was to write a short story based entirely upon
this decision, and on the consequences for a girl whose life might be altered by
the cut. *Bernice Bobs her Hair* was published in 1920. The bob terminated
her story, for with it she was an ugly girl, yet she had captivated her male
audience for a week with the promise of bobbing her hair. Bernice assures the
callow youths that she intends to be a society vampire and that a bob is the
necessary equipment of one. In spite of her secret qualm that bobbing was
unladylike, Bernice claimed to powder her face; probably with the new tinted
face powder which had supplanted the white rice powder of pre-war years.

The great impetus for cheap cosmetics for the multitude was the growth of
the chain store. Before this, most shops had a class system, except for those in
small towns: a girl could hardly venture into Harrods or Bonwit Tellers and
search for cosmetics on their exclusive counters; Selfridges had attempted to
sell cosmetics to the masses but they were still a middle- and lower-middle class
store which attempted to woo suburbia, and the housewives, rather than their
maidservants. When Woolworths opened in Britain and the Five and Ten in
the States, they made cosmetics a certainty for many girls who were apprehensive about them; products and prices could be inspected, and a cheerful
anonymity made these stores more alluring.

They had the right approach for the appetites of the time, as self-service stores would have later for the urban working-class housewife who had never had the money or the experience to face the daunting grey-overalled gentlemen in the affluent grocery shops. The assistants in 'Woolies' were advisers and confederates to the girl with little money and immense ambition.

The upper classes in Britain maintained the mask of their income group which was unique in cosmetics. The 'twenties face, portrayed by later generations, is imagined as a creation of the cinema. In fact, although the elegant maquillage was common in the theatre, the typical fashionable face was not born on film. Eyebrow-plucking was the beginning, and then a certain method of planting rouge, under the cheekbone rather than on it, so that the face was more aquiline, the mouth was imperious, carefully etched and red, there was no mutation of colour, the mask of white powder, pink cheeks and red lips was incapable of great subtlety. To later generations this face is typified by that of Marlene Dietrich, but it was of earlier vintage. (See page 133.) Michael Arlen, an astute foreign writer, saw the English upper-class face very clearly in *The Green Hat,* his best-selling novel which made him £120,000. Iris Storm and her Hispano-Suiza were two symbols of the age, a woman and a car which became eminent in literature. When he meets her, the narrator is drawn by her painted mouth. It does not repulse him as it would have an earlier novelist, but attracts him as an example of her allure. It is described as 'silk-red' and drooping 'like a flower', his ultimate obeisance, occasioned by her sleep, is not the expected kiss but an application of powder, as he notices that she has a shiny patch on her nose. 'To this I applied a little Quelques Fleurs talc powder on a handkerchief that when she awoke she would not think so ill of herself as I did.'

In spite of this, when she wakes, Iris Storm immediately thinks of powdering her face, and he has to fetch the box from the other room, where he carelessly left it . . . 'the case of white jade and the box of black onyx. She powdered, without interest'. Later in the book, Iris is described as having a mask rather than a face; the hero sees her as a study in contrasts; white face, amethyst eyes, red lips, and the inevitable green hat. The novel may seem banal but it captures certain aspects of the period by its own exaggeration. Iris, passing through London society in her great yellow car, is watched 'as men watch women who are known to have had lovers', yet her extremes of style are not more blatant than those of many women in the same circle, but rather more refined.

A more prosaic comment on make-up was given by Angela Rodaway, born in 1918, who began to make up when she was fourteen, and remembered the cosmetics available for a working girl with little money, who lived in Edmonton in the East End of London. While she was still at school she spent money hard earned in holiday jobs on treasures like nail varnish, and she had her hair done by 'Maison Owide', a local firm which used her for apprentices' practice. As she became older she adventured into other areas of London with her comparatively sophisticated friend Sonia, and she relates the meeting which

Left Advertisement for Elizabeth Arden, 1924

Right Advertisement for Pond's, early 1930s
Advertisements for Pond's cosmetics repeated the old formula of endorsement by a 'society beauty' and used lively copy which readers enjoyed. Inevitably, they would become the subject of satire (see *Punch* cartoon on page 124).

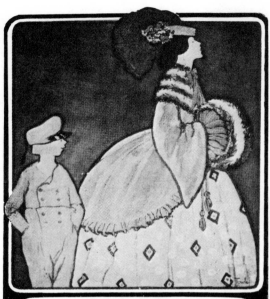

Beauty is built
of many exquisitely perfect details!

AND ELIZABETH ARDEN HAS
DEVOTED SCIENCE AND SKILL TO PERFECTING
EVERY DETAIL OF YOUR FACE AND FORM

The most elaborate *toilette* can be marred by tiny faults of your skin — cheeks that shine, blemishes that flaunt an angry red, coarseness, wrinkles. But each of these faults can be overcome. Not hidden, mind you, but removed! ¶ Elizabeth Arden has developed a scientific treatment to perfect every detail of your appearance. Her method is fundamental: she builds beauty on a sure foundation of firm muscle contours and smooth clear skin. For sallowness, she suggests, not rouge, but stimulating tonics, deftly applied. For wrinkles, not concealing balms, but nourishing skin foods that fill out hollows and attenuations. For coarseness, Elizabeth Arden has developed a wonderful astringent cream that brings the coarsest, laziest pores tightly together, and makes the texture of the skin fine and silky. ¶ The lovely women who follow Elizabeth Arden's method are never dependent upon artifice to create an effect of beauty. If you cannot come to the Arden Salon for personal treatment, you can still achieve wonderful results by caring for your skin at home under Miss Arden's direction. Write to Elizabeth Arden describing the characteristics and faults of your skin, and she will send you a personal letter of advice, outlining the correct treatment for you, and enclosing her book "The Quest of the Beautiful" which describes her method.

Your daily treatment of the skin should include :

Venetian Cleansing Cream — A pure soft cream that melts on the skin, penetrates the pores, dissolves and dislodges all impurities. Supplies the natural oils of the skin, keeps it smooth and supple. Use morning and night and after exposure. . 4/6, 8/6, 12/6.
Venetian Ardena Skin Tonic — Tones, firms and whitens the skin, keeps it clear and radiant. Refreshing and stimulating to the skin. . . . . . . 3/6, 8/6, 16/6.
Venetian Orange Skin Food. — The best deep tissue builder, excellent for a thin, lined or ageing face. Nourishes the skin, keeps it smooth and full. . . . 4/6, 7/6, 12/6.
Venetian Velva Cream. A delicate nourishing cream for full faces. Gives the skin a soft smooth appearance, corrects any tendency to dryness, without fattening. . 4/6, 8/6.
Venetian Special Astringent. For flaccid cheeks and neck. Lifts and strengthens the tissues, tightens the skin . . . . 9/6, 17/6.
Venetian Pore Cream. — Greaseless, astringent cream that closes enlarged pores, corrects their relaxed condition, refines the coarsest skin. . . . . 4/6.
Venetian Muscle Oil. — Feeds and fills out sunken tissues, restores the vitality of impoverished muscles, rounds the contours, smooths the skin. . . . . 4/6, 10/-, 16/6.
Elizabeth Arden's Exercises for Health and Beauty. — Three double-sided gramophone records of exercise movements created especially for women to normalize the weight, stimulate circulation and clear the skin, develop poise and grace . . . . £2 2 0.

ELIZABETH ARDEN

25C, OLD BOND ST.   LONDON W

NEW YORK 673 FIFTH AVENUE   PARIS, 2 RUE DE LA PAIX

CANNES (A.M.) HOTEL ROYAL

The Arden Venetian Preparations are on sale at more than 1,000 smart shops all over the world

---

At 16

MISS ROSE BINGHAM
began using Pond's

Today

as **THE COUNTESS OF WARWICK** *she still follows her girlhood choice*

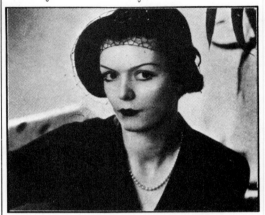

"'I'M SIXTEEN TODAY!' I remember chanting in my bedroom. 'Now what to do to celebrate and show my independence?' Cosmetics were forbidden at school but, after all, I was nearly grown-up and everybody knew Pond's Creams were pure and good for the skin . . . That very afternoon I bought some of the Cold and Vanishing Cream. Going to bed that night, I cold-creamed my face carefully according to the instructions. And in the morning, feeling very guilty, I rubbed a little Vanishing Cream on my nose.

At the end of a week all my friends told me how much better my skin was looking. It felt beautifully soft, too, instead of all rough and flaky.

Ever since that birthday, I've used Pond's Creams regularly and I've never had any trouble with my skin." Here is Lady Warwick's daily beauty care, so simple, it takes only a few minutes of her time ; so inexpensive that every woman can follow it.

" Every night, before going to bed, I spread on plenty of Pond's Cold Cream, leaving it on a few moments so that it softens the skin and sinks deep into the pores. Then I wipe off the soiled cream with Pond's Cleansing Tissues."

There is no purer cream than Pond's, and none that floats out pore-deep dirt so efficiently. That's why skins kept clean with Pond's need never fear blackheads, enlarged pores and blemishes. " Before I powder, and particularly when I am motoring or spending a day in the open, I always use Pond's Vanishing Cream. I find it's easy then to keep my skin soft and fine even in a biting east wind. And, of course, as a powder base, it's unequalled !"

FREE! POWDER OFFER : Write your name and address on the margin of this page, attach a 1d. STAMP to one corner and post in 1½d. sealed envelope to Dept.   , Pond's Extract Company Ltd., Perivale, Middlesex, and we will send you samples of all five shades of Pond's Face Powder : Natural, Peach, Dark Brunette, Rachel 1 and Rachel 2.

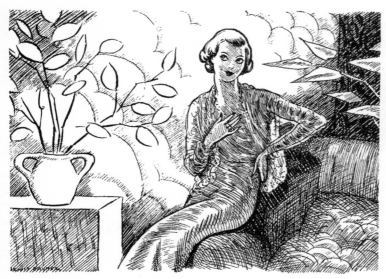

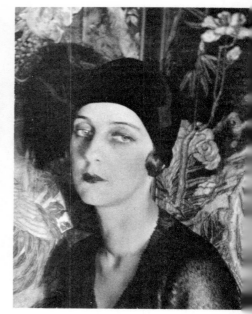

HOW OUR SOCIETY BEAUTIES ARE PHOTOGRAPHED NOWADAYS;
OR, THE COMPOSITE AD.

Evening Frock by Pickins and Bones; Water-wave by Maison Briny;
Complexion by Tintoretto, Ltd.; Manicure by Taloni; Figure by Slim-
Tum Corset Co. Posed by Lady Plantagenet Jones.

Left From *Mr Punch in Mayfair* published 1933
Right Paula Gellibrand photographed by Cecil Beaton, 1930
The inter-war face of the society beauty, with plucked eyebrows, pursed mouth and
an air of hauteur.

inadvertently took place between her bizarre 'Bohemian' and a collection of
earnest Rangers, adult Girl Guides:

The Rangers were all very nice young women, and Sonia and I were going
through an experimental phase, although as far as appearance went, my
experiments were usually more subdued than hers. Sonia was very small so
that she could use brilliant colours, and did. There were two spots of orange
rouge on her cheeks in contrast to the purple lipstick on her wide mouth, and
her eyelids were heavy with emerald shadow under two thin arcs of graphite
masquerading as eyebrows.

Many of these popular cosmetic ideas had come from the United States
directly, as well as by the way of the cinema, for after the Armistice, rich
Americans once more visited Europe and in the interim years when they had
been separated from their ancestral countries by war, they had become in-
involved in styles of decoration which would at first repulse, and then win, the
European women. Visits to Britain were usually en route for France, and in
the matter of dress and cosmetics there was a liaison between America and
France which had been fostered by New York fashion magazines, such as
Vogue, under the direction of Condé Nast. The American girl was much more
involved with make-up than her French or British contemporaries, beauty
parlours were well known in the large cities and most women used powder and
face cream; they even made up in public, displaying a lack of reticence which
would not spread to Britain until the second world war and which is still
unacceptable in some places, so that often even girls who have grown up in the
laissez faire post-war world find it difficult to powder their noses or replace
lipstick in front of other people. The other great innovation from America
was the soft bra. Whalebone had been displaced and now manufacturers were

making a gentler type of foundation, which relied on cut, rather than metal. Clothes were cheaper, owing largely to the synthetic fabric, rayon, which could become the 'poor girl's silk'. Young women, freed from every type of restraint, who lived alone or shared diminutive flats with a female 'chum' were called flappers, and politicians and manufacturers realized that they must be courted in order to make profits in the post-1918 society.

The ideas connected with cosmetics were hectic yet often sensible; in 1915 an American, Maurice Levy, had given licence to the mass production of lipsticks by inventing the metal container, without which they could not have had a nation-wide sale. The notion of colour harmony was exclusive to the richer women who had time to experiment, and who had hopes to differentiate themselves from the working girl by the subtlety of their make-up. One of the new names in the field of cosmetics was Elizabeth Arden, whose salon opened in 1922 in Bond Street. Initially the Arden programme was to save the skin with cream remedies, and as the fashionable treatment of the time involved visits to exclusive little rooms in Mayfair where an elegant woman pampered her face with massage and various tubes of salve, she started using her famous Vienna Youth Masque in her salon. Clients had their features cast in plaster, and from these moulds, padded masks were made for each customer.

During beauty sessions Gland Cream was utilized, which was to be a precursor of the Elizabeth Arden Special Hormone Cream. This was not the only treatment however, each skin was treated for its particular problem with special lotions and the final result was a range of creams with special application which were packaged for the market.

During this decade Professor Burchett was still tattooing. In partnership with a beauty specialist, he had opened a salon at 141 Bond Street, in 1920. Three years later the tomb of an Egyptian princess was opened at Luxor; she had tattoos on her neck, shoulders and breasts, and it became fashionable for English women to have similar tattoos, usually of small insects, engraved on their skin. This practice was even commemorated in a popular song in 1927 which was a skit on Austen Dobson's poem *The Ladies of St. James's*.

The original read:

The Ladies of St James's	But Phillida, my Phillida!
They're painted to the eyes;	Her colour comes and goes,
Their white it stays forever,	It trembles to a lily,
Their red it never dies.	It wavers to a rose . . .

The satirical song echoed in refrain:

From London, Glastonbury, Pondicherri too
Come maids of pale complexion to acquire a ruddier hue,
For lip so pale and brow like snow
Have vanished from the 'comme il faut'
And alabaster's quite de trop
Huzza for the face Tattoo
Huzza for the face Tattoo!

The 'thirties was the period of the rich bitch, brittle ladies who figured in Evelyn Waugh's novels; their ascendancy in London created powerful beauty salons, where gossip could be meted out while thin women were thumped to

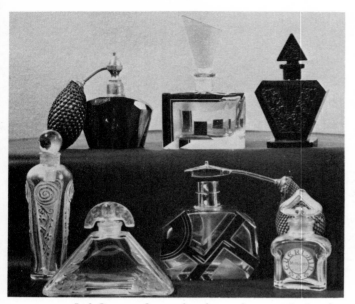
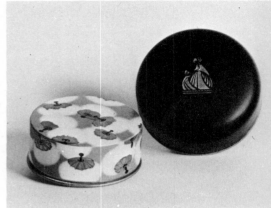

Left Group of scent bottles and sprays dating from 1920 to 1930
Right Coty powder box designed by René Lalique; Lanvin powder box designed by
Madame Jeanne Lanvin

even smaller dimensions. Mingled with the beauty parlours with foreign
sounding names, were a few genuine medical centres where serious skin
conditions could be dealt with vigorously. Medicine was still not a potent force
in make-up as we can see from the advertising of the age. Pond's issued a famous
series of newspaper advertisements which relied on society beauties to state
their preference for Pond's Cold Cream and Pond's Vanishing Cream; the
latter was an early version of tinted foundation cream, and was pale pink.

The packaging of cosmetics in the 'thirties was one of the interesting developments in design. The famous Coty patterns of powder puffs in orange, black
and white which were designed by Lalique; the Yardley perfumes with
charming idiosyncratic flower illustrations owing much to the Art Nouveau
conceptions of Alphonse Mucha; the Lanvin boxes which remained in the
style of the 1920s for many years, and which sensibly rejected more garish,
less identifiable packages, all these made the counters of department stores
bright and alluring. There was a remarkably small variety of shades available
for customers. Lipstick was red, and rouge was red or a slightly hysterical shade
of orange. This tangerine-based colour was the symbol of the 1930s when the
perfume which many women used was Californian Poppy, it was one of the
early success of propaganda, and although it hardly suggested exoticism or
sexual appeal, it resulted from, or in, a rapid 'poppy' fashion, in which heavy
orange flower heads were used for dress and curtain fabrics, made up into silk
flowers which were worn on black satin tea-gowns, and repeated in the colour
of the wearer's lips and rouge; the flower symbol was even incorporated in the
packaging of the period. Perfumes of the years between the wars are curiously
evocative of the age, almost as much as their bottles, which owed more debt
than was ever acknowledged to the glass designs of Lalique and Vernet.

Shalimar dating from 1916 and Mitsouko (1919) promised some of that
liberation which women sought after the first world war; they were based on
essences which made them musky, sensual and sophisticated; the lavender
waters of earlier generations had been discarded in favour of scents and cosmetics which promised sexual success; the overt statement of this was new in

the history of make-up.

The innocent charm of advertising between the wars, clumsy with its over-long blurbs and hints of imagined delights, is understandable when one appreciates that it was not aimed at an over-sophisticated market, but at the girls from factories and domestic service to whom cosmetics were available for the first time.

During the 1939–45 war, cosmetics were in short supply, the promise of a lipstick and a pair of stockings made many US 'airmen more interesting to the girls in the previously occupied parts of Europe, and in Britain country women sometimes resorted to old books in attempts to create lotions which they could not buy. In spite of the conditions of war in Europe it was amazing how many women had hoarded cosmetics in the years before and could make them last for five years. The unfortunates were those who were adolescent, and who had no basic stocks to rely on. In the United States cosmetics were still made and were considered morale boosters, but in Britain and Germany, two European countries which were able to order their own resources, the war effort entailed the shutting down of many small factories, and the larger ones were detailed to produce less superficial goods while the campaign for necessary supplies continued. In Britain, even in those factories which could manufacture cosmetics, output was restricted by the Limitation of Supplies Order of 1940 which cut the usual materials available for cosmetics to twenty-five percent of its pre-war figure. Petroleum and alcohol, two basic ingredients of many cosmetics, were diverted into war supplies, yet what could still be made was sold immediately, creating another interesting irony, that at a time when they were restricted, lipstick, powder and face cream were most desirable and most experimentation was carried out, in preparation for the post-war period, by firms whose stocks were sold as soon as they appeared, and who realized that the actual lack of cosmetics during the war would result in a phenomenal boom afterwards.

Many of the old-established manufacturers were determined that the quality of their products should not fall in the general attempt to substitute ingredients; and owing to this ambition a new attitude to cosmetics arose. This was involved with 'purity', a demand which had often been lacking in earlier periods; and which was associated with increased education, which would lead to the inquisitive shopper. After the war it gave an advantage to those manufacturers who were old-established, and in the upper price ranges of the market. Yardley, Elizabeth Arden, Helena Rubinstein, and the French manufacturing companies became associated with 'quality', an elusive and hitherto disregarded attribute.

In a lower price range, Pond's had the same appeal, and this schism in attitudes to cosmetics was to have interesting repercussions in the years after the war, when the 'lady' would adhere to the products which were considered pure, while the young girl, buying for the first time in an open market, would be attracted by those cosmetics which were less concerned with purity, and more with the actual advantages of imagined sin. In Britain, the Concentration of Industries scheme entailed that manufacturers co-operated to produce their multifarious products under one roof; and the consequence was seen in Yardley, who had moved their factory to Borehamwood in 1939; at the end of the war, less than forty-five percent of their output was under the name of

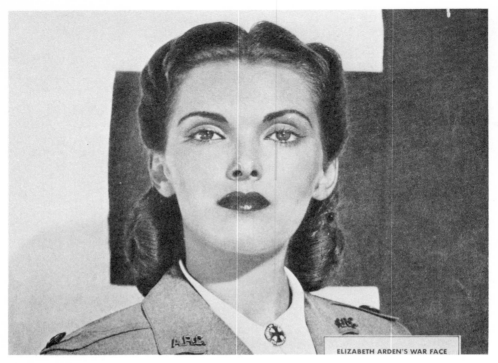

ELIZABETH ARDEN'S WAR FACE

Disguised as a wartime feature (in the *Saturday Evening Post*) Elizabeth Arden advertised the war face, determined, almost hard in fact; it is interesting to see that 'the windblown look is back' and 'her muscles are well trained'.

Yardley, the rest being distributed under the trade-names of Morny, Rosemarine Manufacturing Company, Saville Perfumes and Zenobia. Concurrently, they were doing war work for Crookes Laboratories. In 1942 part of their premises were requisitioned for munitions. Similar stories were true of other large cosmetic factories in Britain.

Owing to propaganda and availability, the American manufacturers had a head start after the war. While the war was on, the American film star achieved more influence than any society beauty. Clara Bow had been the first of many beautiful women who were projected on the screen; during years of shortages and boredom, the faces of Greta Garbo, Veronica Lake, Claire Trevor, Marlene Dietrich, Rita Hayworth and Betty Grable dominated the public appreciation of attractive women. Some of these sirens with highly cosmeticized faces, were now in colour, and although women had been aware of their singular beauty in black and white, the advent of colour films made more impact on cosmetics than has ever been estimated. Previously, the outline of make-up had been seen and viewers had known how to dress their hair in floppy bangs, and the correct shape of a cupid's bow mouth, they knew how to pluck their eyebrows, and all these imitations of celluloid reality needed no more than home aids, such as curlers, tweezers and a contorted face, but with the success of colour films many women throughout the world saw with dismay that the shape of cosmetics was not enough without the exact shades of red which were necessary to emulate Deanna Durbin's or Joan Crawford's lips. The Hollywood cosmetician responsible for many of the changes in coloured cosmetics was Max Factor. As the creator of 'make-up for the stars', this organization had unique attractions for the European women, who had been excluded from the spectrum of shades in make-up. They opened a London

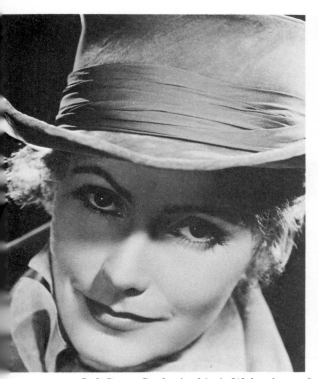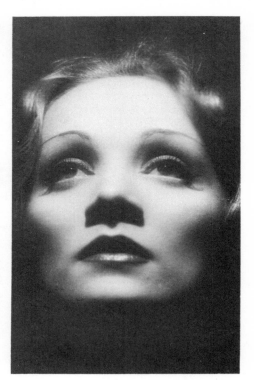

Left Greta Garbo in *Marie Walewska* 1938
Right Marlene Dietrich in *Shanghai Express* 1932
Film stars were the main influence on cosmetics in the 'thirties and 'forties.

salon in 1936. However, many commentators felt that the colours which became current owing to the influence of Hollywood were garish and crude.

Glossy lips may have been treated with glycerine for the cameras but in real life they could be imitated with 'satinized' lipstick—this luminous glow, manufactured very successfully by Lancôme in Paris, gave an eager 'licked' appearance to the lips, and allied with the vivacious colours of the time, made some women of the late 1940s appear like ravening wolves or vampires. These unflattering comparisons came, of course, from the more ladylike members of society who used make-up with such restraint that all the shades from the high-class manufacturers might have been unnoticed, as they were smeared on with such apparent casualness that women of the period appear paralytic in old photographs; for it was not genteel to etch to the corners of one's mouth, while a dislodged blot of colour, largely deleted with a flannel after it had been applied, was quite *comme il faut*. These aspirations to be colourless were not the aims of the *most* elegant women; or of the young factory girls who were unerringly accurate, if unsubtle, in their use of make-up.

The plethora of new scents also resulted in their antithesis, a complete lack of perfume, except for the hardy results of soap, among British middle-class women. At this time they felt that new perfumes covered up worse body smells and the art of true cleanliness was to smell of nothing at all. Fortunately the section of society with this reasoning dwindled during the 'fifties, to such an extent that one large business was built on new perfumes alone. Previously this would have been impossible, for nearly all the perfumes had been by-products of large cosmetic houses, or else from firms which were well-established in the early years of the century. The unusual story of Goya was a legend of the 'fifties. Douglas Collins had founded his firm in 1937 and had

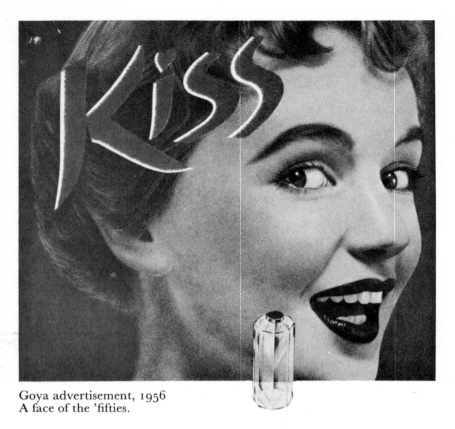

Goya advertisement, 1956
A face of the 'fifties.

left it to serve in the war. It had been a back-parlour project, but when he was demobilized in 1945, Collins put all his savings and his 'demob' money into an old brewery building in Buckinghamshire and seriously worked on the foundation of a new perfume industry. Until that time scents were divided into the outrageously cheap, which were sold in chain stores in vivid bottles, and which turned sour very swiftly; and the alarmingly expensive, which came from France and were restricted by taste as well as price, to the rich. It is doubtful if a provincial girl of either rich or poor family had ever heard of any good perfume, except for Chanel Number Five which had become a byword for worldly sophistication. Her only resort was to the cheap perfumes, and these often heralded their presence by their acrid smell.

Yardley had some of the middle-income market with attractively packaged perfume, but they were so 'safe' that they did not attract a young woman who associated Bond Street and Freesia with her mother. Collins sold reputable perfumes at a low price, made possible by the small amount of perfume available in each bottle, and of good quality. It was well packaged and for many women it was their first opportunity to learn more about perfume. Its very attraction lay in its size, for the handbag phial was not well known before, and the good French perfumes still appeared in dressing table sizes, often in a box which incorporated a stand as well. This experiment was successful, and Goya's Black Rose and Passport perfumes were highly popular; proving that an English manufacturer could break into a field which had previously been largely that of the French cosmeticians. During the 'fifties many attempts were made to imitate his success, and small cosmetic houses, often relying on individual packaging and on exclusiveness (which meant high prices) tried to compete with the titanic businesses which had been set up at the turn of the century, and many failed. By the 1950s the colossal complexes of Max Factor, Helena Rubinstein, Yardley and Elizabeth Arden had control of a major part of the richer market, and the cheaper ranges were catered for by firms like Pond's. The real profit was to be in cosmetics for young girls, and those manufacturers who based their predictions on this market were to succeed. There was little competition for the 'big names' were concerned with older women and were offering 'quality', basing their advertising on their face creams rather than on the decorative cosmetics.

Like Goya, the firm of Gala had been immobilized by the war. At the end of it they were manufacturing three lipstick shades but they projected them in a unique way by using fantasy in their names.

The names of lipsticks had been neglected in the past, and the shade colours of most cosmetics had been restricted to such undescriptive terms as 'rachel', 'dubarri' or 'dark red'. Gala, usurping the young girls' market, introduced Lantern Red and Sea Coral with effective advertising. In 1957 they increased their appeal to younger buyers with Lipline: a pencilled lipstick which was intended to prove easy to handle and firm in outline, it was also one of the first interchangeable lipsticks. Older women had used brushes to spread colour evenly, but like much accurate maquillage, this was a practice for the richer woman with time and patience. During the mid-'fifties many new ideas in cosmetics were promoted by Gala, they recognized the fashion for whiter lips when Italian and French cosmeticians put titanium in their products to produce a pale gleam, and these frosted colours were extended to nail varnishes, including green and silver.

At the end of the 'fifties many colours were co-ordinated, usually under the auspices of *Vogue* who would introduce a seasonal colour and by the resultant publicity persuade manufacturers to produce suitable clothes and cosmetics. Gala's Sari Peach was one of the shades which was developed, with matching and co-ordinating clothes and accessories.

In 1959 Gala introduced a new inexpensive concept in their face powder which had previously been based on two primary shades of yellow or pink. The idea of 'mink' was instantly successful, produced in shades for the English skin which de Grammont had commented on in the seventeenth century as being at its most delightful when it was brown. Many other manufacturers had been experimenting in the same way, but Gala was aiming at the younger market, a type of customer who had not existed before and who would not have understood the subtleties of brown or grey shades before the late 1950s. These avant-garde colours had logical sequels, for women with restricted incomes became less obsessive about blatant cosmetics and turned towards paler and less determinate shades. It was a final proof of the conquest of the subdued colours when Woolworth's stocked delightful pale shades in the early 1960s. These sophisticated shades were once only obtainable at high cost in Paris, from the shade cards of Dior, Orlane and Lancôme; but the colours of Miner's were almost identical and at a fraction of the cost. They also had gimmicky names, daringly suggesting the further emancipation of the young; and they were intended for the many girls who could not afford more than a small sum on a Saturday morning, Like Naked, a pale beige lipstick which made the lips more pale instead of more pink, was to encourage them to use 'barefaced' make up by the end of the decade. The 'total' look came into being slowly and for some

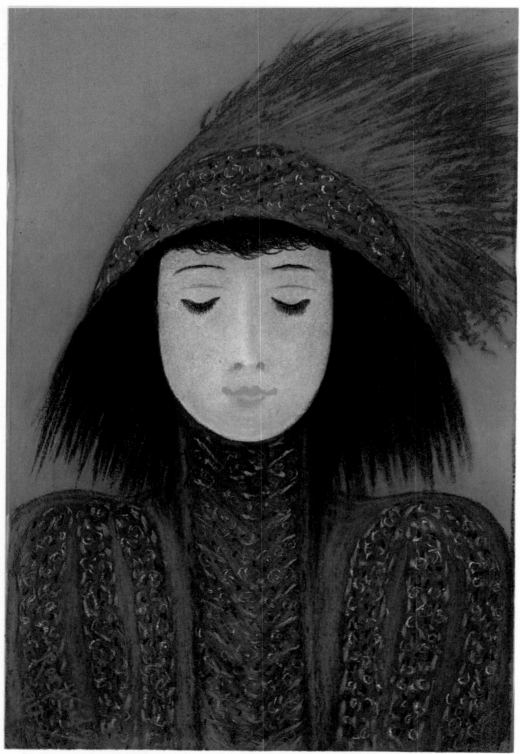

Costume design for head-dress in the style of the Russian Ballet, early 1920s(?)
Author's collection. The brilliant colours of the Russian Ballet on its arrival in Paris
in 1910 revolutionized western European fashions in dress and make-up.

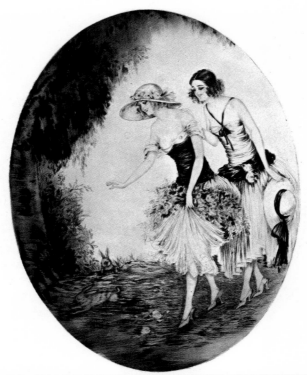

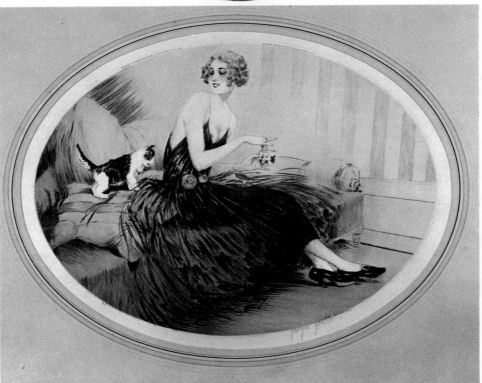

Prints by Audré *above* and Grillet *below* from the series 'Estampes Modernes' 1924.
Author's collection
The chocolate-box prettiness of the early 'twenties becomes almost sinister.

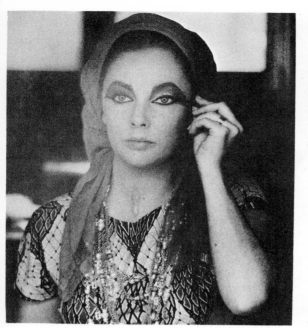
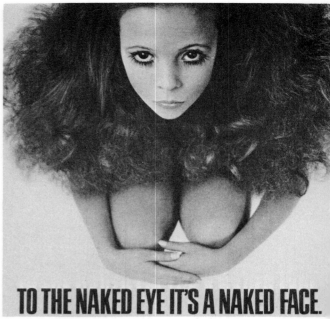

TO THE NAKED EYE IT'S A NAKED FACE.

Left The Cleopatra look became fashionable in the 'fifties when Vivian Leigh made the face of an Egyptian beauty alluring. Later (1961-2) Elizabeth Taylor was to play the same role; and here she puts on make-up to a design dictated by Nefertiti.

Right Advertisement for Mary Quant, designed by Tom Wolsey, 1968

people, not at all. Ten years before, a lipstick which was paler than red was considered eccentric. In 1967 and 1968 the appearance of fashionable women suggested that their faces were as devoid of colour as the faces of medieval saints; a closer inspection showed that the art of make-up had become so rarified that it needed even more time and money than the cruder coloured face of the 'thirties. Lancôme's palette of brown and beige eye shadows in the early 'sixties had forecast an enormous range of browns, creams, whites and greys. The 'Cleopatra' look, with black silky hair, long eyes, elongated with the scientifically designed eye liner, and red lips, had vanished and in its place was a creature who had the innocence of childhood, established by the most involved cosmetic procedure in the history of make-up.

Owing partly to a desire to be different, and partly to a necessity on the part of some cosmetic manufacterers to win young girls from the notion that the 'no make-up' look might terminate with no make-up, some magazines attempted to reinstate the 1940s look, following the fashion for old films and old clothes. In spite of feeble acclamation for the faces of the old Hollywood stars, for vibrant red lipstick and plucked eyebrows, it hardly impinged on the besetting passion for the paler face. Accustomed to soft colour and sombre appearance, the women in the 'sixties would not spend time or money on a maquillage which made them look harder and older. The 1940s look might return in dress, but not in make-up.

It was in advertising rather than ingredients that the make-up of the 'sixties betrayed its period. Previous publicity had been earnest, even dull, with lengthy descriptions of the quality of the product, but in an increasingly egalitarian society there was even more emphasis on the sexual aspect of cosmetics. A comparatively staid business house like Innoxa proclaimed its new lipstick colours in the late 'fifties as: 'EXCITEMENT is as exciting as its name

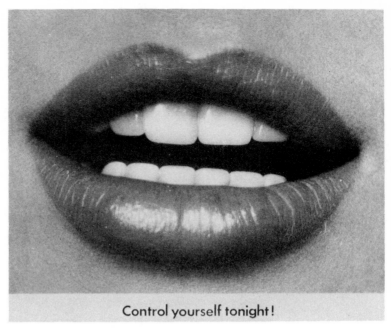

Control yourself tonight!

Advertisement for Germaine Monteil, 1967
The 'daring' caption

and the pillar box brilliance of POSTMAN'S KNOCK just asks to be kissed'. The promise of these captions extended into the 'sixties with copy such as 'things happen to you when you use Badedas' suggesting that even a bubble bath might heighten one's sensual attraction. Innuendoes flowed freely with catch phrases maintaining that one should not play with fire if one did not wish to be burnt, and the general advantages of cosmetics were implicit—bed followed the sight of a new lipstick. Perfume advertisements could play much more with erotic imagery, as did the sequences of photographs showing a lipstick as a phallic object, caressed by the user rather than applied to the mouth (although even this action had its own erotic impact).

The prime cosmetic of the decade was eye shadow. It was to be developed in mascara, eye liner and various other gadgetries connected with the eyes. A top model would take half an hour to decorate her eyes and at the end of that time all the onlooker would see would be misty and muted.

If the inclination to use bright red lipstick was hardly more than the passing phase of a season, women did wish to experiment with colour, although they were more interested in new colours than in a return to the old one. Several manufacturers presented lilac, green and silver lipstick which became allied with the pale pinks and whites so that girls blended their own shades. The do-it-yourself cosmeticians were as prevalent as the do-it-yourself decorators and the varying shades of colour gave them an opportunity to express some individuality at a time when even avant-garde fashion was stereotyped and predictable. There was an increased interest in the.actual formation of the face which had not been seen accurately since the fifteenth century. In an attempt to give bones more prominence, 'blush-ons' came on to the market.

Many manufacturers made them, but Revlon gave them wide publicity. The more expensive products of this type necessitated extra outlay for a large sable brush, but the more elegant and venturous women did not mind buying this in order to brush their Estée Lauder or Germaine Monteil powder on to their cheeks. The cheaper products came with a pad, but both expensive and cheaper brands were often finally applied with a piece of cotton wool. It was ironic that 'blush-ons' as Revlon called them, should be most popular with the twenty to thirty year olds, exactly that generation which would have despised rouge, the closest earlier approximation to the new cosmetic. The variance lay in the method of use for cheeks had been reddened artificially with rouge, but with 'contour' colour, the propagandists insisted that the elemental bone structure was underlined. It was applied on the forehead, the lower cheek cavities, and the chin.

It was almost inevitable that the sequel should be colour to fill in those parts of the face which were not affected by powder or by applied 'contouring', and white eyeshadow cream was introduced. Originally it was intended to deline-ate the cavity above the eye but many women use it on the upper cheekbones too, to erase lines and give extra depth to the face. Before it appeared, a few innovators were using white lipstick on their eyesockets. This had been marketed at a time when red lipsticks were giving way to paler colours, and it had been one of the first do-it-yourself cosmetics. As lipstick colours were refined, many women utilized the left-over white lipsticks on their eyes, although cosmeticians advised them against it; white eye shadow was an example, rare in cosmetic marketing, of customer influencing manufacturer.

This passion for doing things at home, had already led many women to experiments in hair styling at home: The home 'perm', tongs, and colour tinting applied from a packet, culminated in electric rollers, portable hair dryers, and the universal acceptance of the wig, which would once have been a sad necessity for a bald woman, but now was a cosmetic necessity for models who had to vary their appearance with every picture. The general public seized on the idea of wigs; they were initially a badge of affluence, and as their prices dropped with the introduction of synthetic hair, they were treated as objects for fun rather than serious consequence, and after using them to hide unclean or unkempt hair or relieve the tedium of genuine colour or length, many women relegated them to the back of the cupboard. This mentality was one of the symbols of the 'sixties, especially in the United States and Britain. The cosmetic users were younger than they had ever been, lipsticks were used by girls of eleven and twelve who wore make-up with the audacity of twenty year olds, they had large allowances from parents who were, said some critics, compensating for their own lack of interest in their children. Spurred by television, advertising campaigns and films to be unnaturally precocious, many young girls were able to spend a fair sum per week on adornment, and the bulk of their money went on cosmetics and stockings, the cheapness of cosmetics, and their easy availability, demanding little decision-making in the weekend hours when the shops were open. The Saturday morning shopper was 'teen and pre-'teen in age and the department and chain stores were concerned with baiting her. She was easily caught with every new shade and package.

Older women found that frustrations of money, daily routine and household chores were most easily smoothed with the eyeshadow case or a new lipstick. They were cheap, a matter of a few shillings or a dollar, and this assured the victim of advertising that she was not guilty of extravagance. She was buying something definable in a way that a bar of chocolate or a bunch of flowers could never be. The small cosmetic represented adventure, glamour and high living at a low price. It is also true to say that as a panacea for the ills of married

afford it, and if one cared to have it done. It was often a rich woman's whim and it was also discernible after a certain time by the straitened action of the muscles. Tired muscles could not be moved from the face, but the cosmetic surgeon did remove some of the wrinkled skin, and that which was left was pulled into smoothness. In face-lifting forehead wrinkles are removed by taking a crescent of skin from the hair so that the resultant scar is covered when the hair grows again. There was some disparity between making the incision on the hairline, or behind it, as a noted German surgeon, Doctor Joseph, maintained that there was no benefit gained from covering the scar with the possibly dirty hair. Concealing the scar is the most important problem in cosmetic surgery; the incision is usually made at a place parallel to the wrinkles but in a position in which it will not intrude.

Lips can be moderated by making a wedge-shaped incision in them and removing the centre of an over-large lip; even hare lips can be corrected by plastic surgery if the patient is submitted as a child. Obtrusive ear lobes can be cut down in size, and jaws can be made more or less determined by building up the jaw line or removing excess bone.

Noses are the most usual problem for the plastic surgeon. The shape is often dependent on the growth of cartilage, and this can be removed. A nose with a wide bridge can be altered by fracturing the bones and fixing them together again. Nostrils and tips of noses can be altered with the same, or similar techniques, of deletion and addition. Cosmetic surgery benefited incalculably from the war, when burnt or damaged men were knit together again and skin grafts and new parts of faces and bodies left very little sign of the operation afterwards. Later, cosmetic surgery would be used to aid the unfortunates who had sex-change problems and wished to make their bodies and faces conform to the accepted mode for men or women. However surgery has become less common for the fashionable woman. Stories in newspapers occasionally attribute the success of pop-singers or actors to operations on their faces, but the general public care less for conformity and unless the face is absolutely unsightly few young people worry about the size of their nose or the lobes of their ears. Occasionally a doctor might advise surgery if a patient were becoming neurotically obsessed with an affliction but the problem is more often an emotional than a physical one.

Emotions have also played a part in changing attitudes towards male cosmetics. Before the 'sixties, men were expected to be almost aggressively masculine. Their cosmetics were limited to after-shave lotions which had all the aura of the great outdoors. As softer, more colourful clothes came into their wardrobes there was less pressure on men to be overtly masculine, and it is now absolutely advantageous for a man to smell of some scent which does not have immediate connotations with the sea or country life. Imported perfumes from France and the United States have become more and more heterosexual: Moustache, Eau de Vetiver, Habit Rouge and Eau Sauvage are all appealing for women as well as men. These charming, fragrant and urbane perfumes are expensive, but the mass-market manufacturers appreciate that they are more sophisticated than those popular colognes redolent of tobacco and leather; even the most popular toiletries have become more astringent. The selling force of complementary-scented lotions had been successful in the female field and the corresponding idea of male ranges of cosmetics was pioneered by

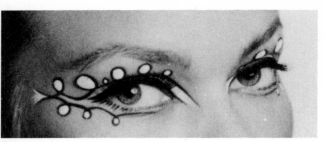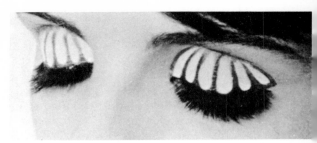

Fantasy eye make-up by Pablo of Elizabeth Arden, mid-1960s

Helena Rubinstein, who introduced the Prince Gourielli range in honour of her husband. This habit of extending one smell through a sequence of lotions is immensely advantageous for the Christmas gift trade, which persecutes the public with boxed cosmetics, half of which will not be used by the recipient of the present; however the idea has never really extended to France where most men are contented with one lotion to do the work of the several categorized for the English and American market.

The next major development in cosmetics will almost certainly be intended for men. Initially it will be in the field of the fast suntan and already the market is being explored with this lotion, beginning with sexy advertising for He Tan. From this, will develop the suntan which is smeared on to the body as a cream and which appears in a few hours as swift all-over colour. It is used already by many men, but the appeal to them has only been tentative; the general advertising slant is towards women.

The 'queer' societies in the countries of northern Europe have made cosmeticized men repulsive to the sensitively masculine societies of the United States and Britain; however this may be because they have attempted to emulate the female's more colourful maquillage, which is unsuitable in male make-up. The more promising market will be in lotions to induce various shades of brown, blended with a paler brown lipstick.

Old photographs of matinée idols display them as aggressively red-lipped, yet the natural trait for men should be to have paler mouths, well delineated, and the 'lip-line' type of dispenser will be more useful for them than for women. Another fault in attempts to cosmeticize men has been plucked eyebrows, which are associated with effete actors of the 'thirties: in the future, men may find that it is more charming to display heavy but well-shaped eyebrows, plucked to a distinctive shape, and then crayoned in with dark grey pencil. Pale nail lacquer should become almost obligatory as it will be complemented by sunburnt hands.

There will be little competition with women: in many ways the cosmetics of husband and wife will correspond and they can share their palette. If women find the idea of male colour, or of a heightening of natural colour, too intimidating or too boring, they may consider the more extravagant recent movements towards patterned faces and bodies in the manner of primitive men, or the use of elaborate decoration above and below the eye. Designs may be appliquéd with mock tattoos, which are actually transfers in different colours which can be washed off in a bath in the evening. These witty but complicated ideas may never become truly popular; in a period when time is perpetually scarce, most women will use the least problematical cosmetics. The banishment of smoke and even of petrol fumes might give a new impetus to the natural look as the skin will need less protective barriers, and only a nourishing cream at night. It will be ironic if we return to the position of the early-eighteenth-century extremists, and men are finally more cosmeticized than women.

Bibliography

Aldburgham, Alison *Shops and Shopping* 1964 Allen & Unwin, London

Aldburgham, Alison *View of Fashion* 1966 Allen & Unwin, London

Aldred, Cyril *The Egyptians* 1961 Thames & Hudson, London; Praeger, New York

Apuleius trans. Robert Graves *The Golden Ass* 1950 Penguin, Harmondsworth; and 1951 Farrar, Straus & Giroux, New York

Arlen, Michael *The Green Hat* 1968 Cassell, London

Aubrey, John ed. L. Dick *Brief Lives* 1962 Penguin, Harmondsworth; and 1963 University of Michigan Press

Ayer, Harriet Hubbard *Beauty, A Women's Birthright* 1904 Pond's, London, New York

Ayer, Margaret Hubbard and Isabella Taves *Three Lives of Harriet Hubbard Ayer* 1957 W. H. Allen, London

Beaton, Cecil *The Glass of Fashion* 1953 Weidenfeld & Nicolson, London; and Doubleday, New York

Binder, Pearl *Muffs and Morals* 1953 Harrap, London

Bleackley, Horace *The Story Of A Beautiful Duchess* 1907 Constable, London

Bloom, Ursula *The Elegant Edwardian* 1954 Hutchinson, London

Bryant, Arthur *The Age of Elegance* 1954 Collins, London

Burchett, George *Memoirs of a Tattooist* 1958 Oldbourne, London

Burton, Elizabeth *The Elizabethans at Home* 1958 Secker & Warburg, London

Burton, Elizabeth *The Jacobeans at Home* 1962 Secker & Warburg, London

Burton, Elizabeth *The Georgians at Home* 1964 Longmans Green, Harlow

Campbell, Joseph *Masks of God* 1960 Secker & Warburg, London

Chapman, Hester W. *Lady Jane Grey* 1962 Jonathan Cape, London

Chateaubriand trans. Robert Baldick *Memoirs* 1961 Penguin, Harmondsworth

Cook, James ed. J. Barrow *Voyages of Discovery* 1967 Everyman, London

Coulton, G. C. *Medieval Scene* 1959 Cambridge University Press; and Peter Smith, Magnolia, Mass.

Cunnington, C. Willett *Handbook of English Costume in the Sixteenth Century* 1956 Faber & Faber, London; and 1962 Hillary, New York

Cunnington, C. Willett *Handbook of English Costume in the Seventeenth Century* 1955 Faber & Faber, London; and Hillary, New York

Cunnington, C. Willett *Handbook of English Costume in the Eighteenth Century* 1957 Faber & Faber, London; and 1966 Hillary, New York

Cunnington, C. Willett *Handbook of English Costume in the Nineteenth Century* 1966 Faber & Faber, London; and Hillary, New York

Darwin, Charles *The Voyage of the Beagle* 1961 Everyman, London; and 1962 Doubleday, New York

D'Assailly, Gisele *Ages of Elegance* 1968 Macdonald, London

Davis, Dorothy *A History of Shopping* 1966 Routledge & Kegan Paul, London; and University of Toronto Press

Desroches-Noblecourt, Christianne *Tutankhamen* 1963 The Connoisseur and Michael Joseph, London; and 1965 Doubleday, New York

Dodds, John W. *The Age of Paradox* 1953 Gollancz, London

Doughty, Charles M. ed. Edward Garnett *Passages from Arabia Deserta* 1931 Jonathan Cape, London; and Peter Smith, Magnolia, Mass.

Dumas, F. Ribadeau *Cagliostro* 1968 Allen & Unwin, London; and Grossman, New York

Elliot, Blanche B. *A History of English Advertising* 1962 Batsford, London

Eydoux, Henri-Paul *The Buried Past* 1966 Weidenfeld & Nicolson, London; and Praeger, New York

Flaubert, Gustave ed. Francis Steegmuller *Selected Letters* 1954 Hamish Hamilton, London; and Farrar, Straus & Giroux, New York

Fraser, Lady Antonia *Mary Queen of Scots* 1969 Weidenfeld & Nicolson, London; and Dell, New York

Gramont, Sanche de *Epitaph for Kings* 1968 Hamish Hamilton, London

Grimal, Pierre *The Civilisation of Rome* 1963 Allen & Unwin, London; and Simon & Schuster, New York

Hurwood, Bernhardt J. *The Golden Age of Erotica* 1968 Tandem, London; and (as *Erotica*) Paperback Library, New York

Keppel, Sonia *Edwardian Daughter* 1958 Hamish Hamilton, London

Keyes, Jean *A History of Women's Hairstyles 1500 – 1965* 1966 Methuen, London

Kidder, J. E. *Japan before Buddhism* 1959 Thames & Hudson, London; and 1966 Praeger, New York

Kirwan, Daniel Joseph *Palace and Hovel* 1963 Abelard-Schumann, London; and New York

Laver, James *Edwardian Promenade* 1958 Edward Hulton, London

Lindsay, Jack *Leisure and Pleasure in Roman Egypt* 1965 Frederick Muller, London; and 1966 Barnes & Noble, New York

McClure-Thomson, Elizabeth, ed. *The Chamberlain Letters* 1966 John Murray, London; and Putnam, New York

Mitchell, R. J. and M. D. R. Leys *A History of the English People* 1950 Longmans Green, Harlow

Moehr, Ellen *The Dandy* 1960 Secker & Warburg, London

Moorehead, Alan *The Blue Nile* 1962 Hamish Hamilton, London; and Harper & Rowe, New York

Mossiker, Frances *The Queen's Necklace* 1961 Gollancz, London; and Simon & Schuster, New York

Murray, Margaret M. *The Witch Cult in Western Europe* 1963 Oxford University Press; and Peter Smith, Magnolia, Mass.

Myers, A. R. *England in the Late Middle Ages* 1952 Penguin, Harmondsworth

Myknas, George *Ancient Mycenae* 1957 Routledge & Kegan Paul, London

Piper, David *The English Face* 1957 Thames & Hudson, London

Platter, Thomas ed. and trans. Sean Jennett *Journal of a Younger Brother* 1963 Frederick Muller, London; and Dufour, Chester Springs, Pa.

Point, Father Nicolas *Wilderness Kingdom, Indian Life in the Rocky Mountains 1840 – 47* 1967 Michael Joseph, London; and Holt, Rinehart & Winston, New York

Pyne, Captain ed. Warburton *Prince Rupert's Voyage to the West Indies* 1849

Rodaway, Angela *A London Childhood* 1960 Batsford, London

Rowse, A. L. *The England of Elizabeth* 1950 Macmillan, London; and 1961 Collier Macmillan, New York

Rubinstein, Helena *My Life for Beauty* 1965 The Bodley Head, London; and 1963 Simon & Schuster, New York

Sadleir, Michael *Bulwer: a Panorama* 1931 Constable, London

Sitwell, Sir Osbert *Noble Essences* 1950 Macmillan, London

Stanley, Louis *The Beauty of Women* 1955 W. H. Allen, London

Stanton, Doris Mary *English Society in the Early Middle Ages* 1951 Penguin, Harmondsworth

Van-Cles-Reden, Sybille *The Buried People* 1955 Rupert Hart Davies, London

Williams, Neville *Elizabeth I, Queen of England* 1967 Weidenfeld & Nicolson, London and 1968 Dutton, New York

Wilson, John Dover *Life in Shakespeare's England* 1944 Penguin, Harmondsworth

Wykes Joyce, Max *Cosmetics and Adornment* 1961 Peter Owen, London; and Philosophical Library, New York

Also various newspapers and magazines 1700 – 1900; and copies since 1920 of the *Daily Mail, Elle, Esquire, Harper's Bazaar, Ladies' Home Journal, Marie-Claire, Nova, The Observer Colour Magazine, Playboy, Queen, Seventeen, The Sunday Times Colour Magazine, The Times, Twen, Vogue, Woman's Mirror, Woman's Own.*